Techniques of measurement in medicine: 5

Series Editor: Professor ᴾ
Department of Medic
St Bartholomew's Ho.
Consultant Editor: Pr

Instrumentation for co

Instrumentation for coronary care

S.L.GRANDIS

Cambridge University Press

CAMBRIDGE

LONDON   NEW YORK   NEW ROCHELLE

MELBOURNE   SYDNEY

Published by the Press Syndicate of the University of Cambridge
The Pitt Building, Trumpington Street, Cambridge CB2 1RP
32 East 57th Street, New York, NY 10022, USA
296 Beaconsfield Parade, Middle Park, Melbourne 3206, Australia

© Cambridge University Press 1981

First published 1981

Printed in Great Britain at the University Press, Cambridge

British Library Cataloguing in Publication Data
Grandis, S.L.
Instrumentation for coronary care. –
(Techniques of measurement in medicine; 5).
1. Heart – Diseases 2. Critical care medicine
3. Medical instruments and apparatus
I. Title II. Series
616.1'2   RC682   80-49927
ISBN 0 521 23548 0 hard covers
ISBN 0 521 28024 9 paperback

Contents

Preface

Nurses are now involved increasingly with monitoring various parameters of patients both on the general ward and in high dependency areas such as the Coronary Care Unit and the angiography theatre. They are given, and readily accept, responsibility for detecting life-threatening dysrhythmias and treating them in emergencies by giving intravenous therapy such as lignocaine to prevent ventricular fibrillation, and atropine to prevent asystole. The Coronary Care nurse is also often taught to use powerful and potentially hazardous equipment such as the defibrillator.

Many books have been written on dysrhythmias and their treatment. The aim of this book is partly to explain, in simple terms, uses to which machines are put and how to recognize and correct some problems. Hours of anguish are sometimes caused to the nurse trying to obtain a clear trace on a cardioscope, or attempting to record an emergency electrocardiogram for evaluation. Patients can be pestered mercilessly in the hope of achieving a trace worth studying. Artefacts may be misinterpreted, even by medical staff, causing wrong treatment to be prescribed.

An increasing amount of equipment is available for diagnosis and treatment of electrical and pumping problems in the heart. The principles may be basic but usage is made difficult by small sections of the apparatus failing or malfunctioning through inadequate care or ignorance. The machine quickly becomes an enemy rather than a helpful friend. Learning by trial and error has its place, but not when human life is at stake. A little education on correct use and a few simple techniques in troubleshooting will help the nurse to use the equipment effectively and safely, allaying her own fears and helping the patient feel more comfortable, relaxed and confident.

The patient must never be allowed to feel like 'a lump of meat at the end of a wire', as a patient once described himself. The equipment should be thought of as only an aid to excellent treatment and nursing care.

1. Basics

In this book several words or phrases may be used which have come to acquire a specific meaning in cardiology jargon, and some technical words appear which may need further explanation. In this chapter an attempt is made to clarify some of these points.

Also, whilst this chapter does not intend to teach interpretation of electrocardiograms (ECGs), some explanation may be useful for later chapters. It is hoped that this chapter will help to build a foundation for further study for some readers and fill gaps in knowledge for others. There are a few basic principles which help to make looking at ECGs and rhythm strips simpler, more interesting, and which lead to greater understanding.

Conduction of electricity in the heart

The normal heart beat is initiated when electrical activity is transmitted from the sino-atrial (S-A) node in the right atrium and waves of current spread through the right and left atria to the atrioventricular (A-V) node (Fig. 1.1). This current causes atrial depolarization which makes the atria contract (atrial systole), the force of which pushes blood from the atria to the ventricles. The current then passes with a slight delay from the A-V node down the Bundle of His. The ventricles are filling with blood at this stage. When the electricity spreads from the Bundle of His into the Purkinje system the ventricles are depolarized and thus stimulated to contract forcing blood from the right and left ventricles to the pulmonary artery and aorta respectively. This is termed ventricular systole. A short recovery phase follows, called re-

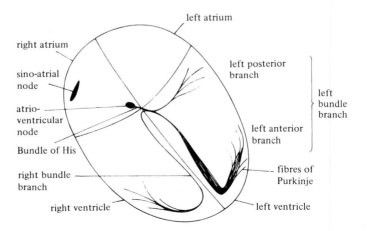

Fig. 1.1. Schematic representation of the conduction system of the heart.

polarization, as the electricity is restabilized in the cells. Next there is a period of inaction while the heart fills, its length dependent on the heart rate. Repolarization and the period of inaction are termed electrical diastole.

Other myocardial cells, apart from those specifically involved in the conducting system, are capable of producing atrial and ventricular depolarization. In the normal heart, the position of a cell in the heart determines the rate at which it can dischrage. The cells at the sino-atrial or pacemaker node are normally the fastest, so the conduction sequence occurs as described above. Cells in the ventricles have a slower intrinsic rate, and will only start their own (idioventricular) rhythm if the impulses from the atria are blocked or absent.

Myocardial damage, drugs or chemical imbalance may make some cells unusually irritable, and so they discharge faster than the S-A node, causing an ectopic beat. If the ectopic beat occurs at a vulnerable time in the cycle, ventricular tachycardia or ventricular fibrillation may result. One ectopic beat may be enough to cause this (Fig. 1.2). It is sometimes a useful phenomenon: if the conducting system fails or the sino-atrial rate is too slow, another focus may cause regular contractions at a good rate. This is termed an 'escape rhythm'.

Normally sodium ions are mainly outside in the extra-cellular fluid and potassium ions are mainly inside in the intra-cellular fluid of each cell. Stimulation of the cell results in a sudden change of the membrane's ability to maintain this balance between sodium and potassium. The resulting flow of sodium into the cell and subsequently potassium out of the cell results in the action potential. This has two major effects: it mobilizes calcium and promotes contraction of the cell; and the ionic currents which produce the action potential stimulate neighbouring cells. If the cell membrane is damaged a leakage of ions increases the chance

Fig. 1.2. Sinus tachycardia followed by a ventricular ectopic beat. A second ventricular ectopic beat (↑) falls on the T wave of the preceding beat resulting in ventricular fibrillation.

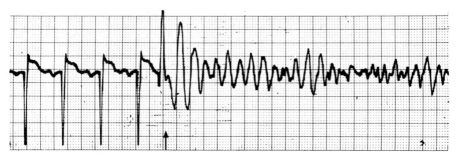

of a premature depolarization or ectopics, and may cause ventricular fibrillation. Many drugs are available to suppress this tendency and a large part of the nurse's responsibility while watching the cardiac monitor, is to spot the beats which are potentially hazardous so that appropriate preventive measures can be taken.

The restabilizing of ions occurs during repolarization, or the T-wave phase. A small part of the T wave, normally from the peak to the bottom of the downward slope, is known as the vulnerable period. This is the time when ectopic activity is most likely to result in ventricular tachycadia or ventricular fibrillation. In disease the vulnerable period may be more extensive.

The electrical currents detected by applying electrodes on different parts of the body, i.e. with a different relationship to the heart, form patterns around a base line (isoelectric line). These can be continuously monitored on a cardioscope from one, two or more directions simultaneously, or a 12 lead ECG can be taken at intervals to demonstrate activity seen in the frontal or horizontal view (see Chapter 2). Each part of the pattern produced by the flow of electric current in the heart is conventionally labelled for clarity (Figs. 1.3 and 1.4). Care must be taken not to confuse a U wave with a T wave or extra P wave.

To describe ventricular depolarization more fully it should be explained that the beginning of the QRS complex records activation of the interventricular septum, followed by the inner layers of both ventricles spreading to the outer surfaces. As the left ventricle has far thicker walls than the right ventricle and because it takes longer to depolarize the left than the right ventricle, left ventricular activation is responsible for the majority of the QRS complex.

Fig. 1.3. ECG terminology. P, waves of electrical excitation (depolarization) causing atrial contraction; Q, R, S, waves of electrical excitation causing ventricular contraction; T, ventricular recovery (repolarization). U, often follows the T wave, it may be normal but it can also indicate electrolytic imbalance, especially hypokalaemia.

Fig. 1.4. Rhythm strip shows prominent U waves. It is important not to confuse the U wave with a T wave especially when ectopic beats follow closely. This is not an 'R on T' ectopic (↑).

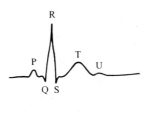

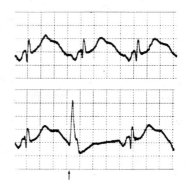

Further terminology is applied to clarify other points. P′ denotes atrial activity arising from other places in the atria apart from the S-A node, e.g. atrial ectopics (Fig. 1.5). The saw-toothed waves produced in atrial flutter are known as F waves (Fig. 1.6). 'Q' is the first deflection following a P wave if it is downward in relation to the baseline, i.e. negative. 'R' is any upward deflection (positive) following a P wave. If there is a second positive deflection it is denoted R′. 'S' is any negative deflection following an R wave.

Capital letters and lower case letters can be used to show relative sizes of parts of the complex. The ventricular systolic part of the complex may be written as Rs to demonstrate that the voltage of the R wave is greater than the S wave (Fig. 1.7).

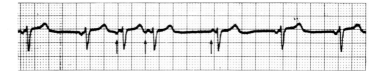

Fig. 1.5. Sinus rhythm with atrial ectopic beats (↑).

Fig. 1.6. Atrial flutter. This enlarged rhythm strip taken in lead V1 demonstrates the characteristic saw-tooth 'F' waves which occur constantly even during ventricular systole (v) and distort the T waves.

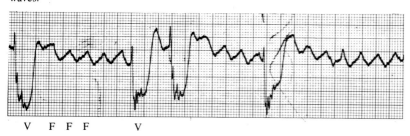

V   F F F   V

Fig. 1.7. Examples showing how large and small letters can be used to show different parts of a wave complex. (a), Rs; (b) Qr; (c) qRs.

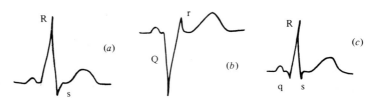

When looking at ECG wave forms it is easier to relate them to the positive electrode only. Electricity flowing towards a positive electrode gives a positive (upward) pattern. Electricity flowing away from a positive electrode gives a negative (downward) pattern. For a given voltage the more directly the electricity flows towards a positive electrode the taller it will be. Conversely the more directly electricity flows away from the positive electrode the deeper it will be. Electricity flowing at 90° to a positive electrode is neither going towards nor away from the electrode and so shows an averaged pattern with very little deflection, usually RS.

Using the information given so far about the flow of electricity in relation to a positive electrode it will be easily seen why a typical negative pattern normally appears in the recording lead V1 of a 12 lead ECG (Chapter 2), assuming normal conduction (Fig. 1.8).

If the positive electrode is placed to the right and above the heart in the position shown in Fig. 3.4, it will be seen that the main flow of electricity in both atria and ventricles is away from it, resulting in a negative pattern. This information can be used when studying ventricular ectopics.

Right ventricular ectopic
The current arises in the right side of the heart and travels towards the left, or away from the positive electrode, giving a negative pattern. This takes longer than travelling through the normal conduction pathway, therefore the QRS complex is wider (Fig. 1.9).

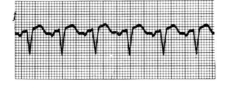

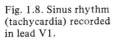
Fig. 1.8. Sinus rhythm (tachycardia) recorded in lead V1.

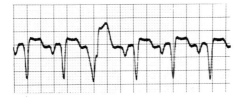

Fig. 1.9. Sinus rhythm with a right ventricular ectopic (V1).

Left ventricular ectopic

The current arises in the left ventricle and travels towards the right, or towards the positive electrode, giving a positive deflection which, again, is wider than normal. In ectopic beats the T wave is usually in the opposite direction to the main wave of the QRS complex (Fig. 1.10). V1 is also useful in diagnosing sinus rhythm with right or left bundle branch block where similar rules apply.

Right bundle branch block

The electricity flows from the A-V node down the intact left bundle and activates the ventricular septum from left to right, i.e. towards the positive electrode, therefore the pattern is initially positive. As the left ventricle is activated, there is a downward deflection (Fig. 1.11). Later the electricity turns to the right ventricle where normal conduction in the right bundle is blocked, moving towards the positive electrode, so the second part of the pattern is positive. The process takes longer than travelling through the normal pathway, therefore the QRS complex is wider than normal (equal to or greater than 0.12 s).

Left bundle branch block

Conversely, when there is total left bundle branch block the current flows from the S-A node down the right bundle and then

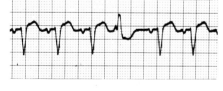

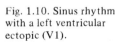
Fig. 1.10. Sinus rhythm with a left ventricular ectopic (V1).

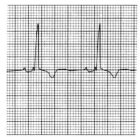

Fig. 1.11. Sinus rhythm with right bundle branch block.

slowly through the left ventricle all away from the positive electrode, producing a negative wide complex in V1 (Fig. 1.12).

Ectopic beats
An ectopic beat is a beat arising from an abnormal source. It is usually premature but may occur later if the basic rhythm is slow, when another focus may take over at a slightly faster rate. Examples of ectopic beats are ventricular, junctional and atrial.

In an atrial ectopic the P' (i.e. the initiating wave) is usually a different shape from the sinus P wave. Sometimes it is difficult to see if it is very premature and is embedded in the previous T wave. The clue to the presence of an atrial ectopic P' may be a distorted T wave compared to the normal beats.

Aberration
When referring to heart beats this implies that the electrical stimulation has taken a different pathway from usual. This often happens following a very early atrial ectopic which occurs during the T wave phase or ventricular repolarization. Stimulation passes from the atria to the A-V node and Bundle of His but finds that the pathway to the ventricles is not completely recovered and therefore not fully able to conduct. The resting part is said to be 'refractory'. Electricity can pass through to stimulate a part of the ventricle immediately, but other parts contract slightly later, giving partial or complete right or left bundle branch block (see Figs. 1.11 and 1.12). This is particularly common during a supraventricular tachycardia when stimulation from the atria is so rapid that the conduction pathways are found to be partially refractory. The resultant complexes may be wide and bizarre and must not be mistaken for ventricular tachycardia as the treatment is different.

At times it is difficult to decide from where a particular beat arises while watching a moving trace on a cardioscope. These are

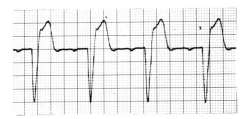

Fig. 1.12. Sinus rhythm with left bundle branch block.

sometimes referred to as 'FLBs' (funny looking beats) until they are identified on the write-out (Fig. 1.13).

Artefact

In ECG terminology this word refers to an extraneous electric impulse which appears on a monitoring screen or on a write-out of a rhythm.

Artefacts may be deliberate such as those produced by a battery-operated pacemaker (see Chapter 5) or the spikes which appear on the ECG trace to demonstrate triggering of an aortic balloon pump (see Chapter 6).

The word artefact most often refers to electrical interference, produced from other electrical devices or from other electrical sources in the body such as skeletal muscle, causing somatic tremor (Fig. 1.14). These distort the trace causing the possibility of misinterpretation of a signal or they make it impossible to interpret at times. Other words used to describe artefact as interference are 'noise', 'shatter' and 'hum'. Correct earthing of electrical equipment helps to abolish it. Battery-run equipment is less prone to such interference. Placement of monitoring electrodes to avoid muscular areas helps to reduce interference (see Chapter 3).

ECG paper. For diagnosis and as a permanent record, cardiac rhythm is written out on ECG paper. ECG paper is divided into squares, for ease of measuring the speed of the trace and the voltages (Fig. 1.15). Standard size paper is used internationally, which travels at speeds that can be altered from the normal 25 mm/s to other variants: 10, 15, 50 and 100 mm/s (Fig. 1.16).

Fig. 1.13. 'FLBs': this is probably a supraventricular tachycardia conducted with aberration, and not ventricular tachycardia, even though the P waves are not evident throughout; the first beat of the run starts with a premature P wave.

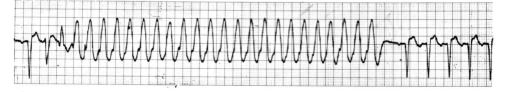

Fig. 1.14. Somatic tremor caused by tensed skeletal muscle produces the interference seen on this rhythm strip.

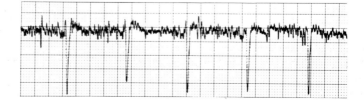

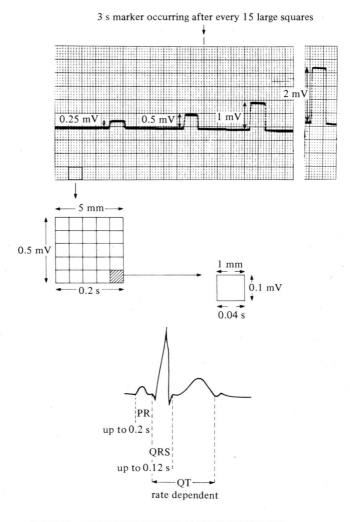

Fig. 1.15. Electro-
cardiographic paper for
measuring time and
voltage, giving linear
response to increasing
calibration deflections.
Note: these figures are
the upper time limits.
The PR interval is
measured from the
beginning of the P wave
to the initial deflection
of the ventricular com-
plex whether it is Q or
R. The QRS interval is
measured from the
initial deflection of the
ventricular complex to
the last deflection. The
QT interval is measured
from the initial deflec-
tion of the ventricular
complex, whether it is
Q or R, to the end of
the T wave.

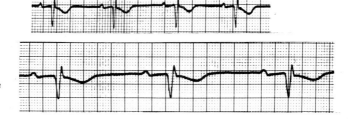

Fig. 1.16. *Top*, Sinus
rhythm recorded at
25 mm/s; *bottom*, same
rhythm recorded at
50 mm/s.

Rate calculation. Using this information the rate on an ECG trace can be calculated. As the paper usually travels at 25 mm/s each millimetre (fine lines) represents 0.04 s. The heavy lines are drawn 5 mm apart and represent 5 × 0.04 seconds (0.2 s). There are 300 heavy lines per minute. To measure ventricular rate, count the number of spaces bounded by heavy lines between two adjacent complexes and divide this number into 300. This method is reasonably accurate if the rhythm is regular.

If the rhythm is irregular a reasonable figure is deduced by counting the number of beats occurring within three seconds (i.e. between sixteen heavy lines). Some paper is marked at 3 s intervals for ease of measurement. Multiply the number within 3 s by 20 to give the rate per minute. If there is a beat at either end count it as a half or quarter for greater accuracy.

ECG rulers are also available for quickly measuring a heart rate on paper recorded at 25 mm/s and 50 mm/s.

Calculating the heart rate from the monitor should never be used as a substitute for feeling the patient's pulse regularly or listening to the heart beat with a stethoscope. A large pulse deficit, due to ineffective beats which may not open the aortic valve, may be present but could be missed. A pulse deficit is often detected when there is an irregular rhythm, e.g. atrial fibrillation. The force of ventricular contraction varies so that occasional weak beats are produced. Usually the faster the ventricular rate the more beats are missed at the radial pulse. Ventricular ectopic beats are often detected at the radial pulse as missed beats as the force of ventricular contraction is not always great enough to be felt in the peripheral arteries. When recording rate, it should be noted clearly on the chart whether it is pulse or heart (i.e. apex) rate. To plot a pulse rate continuously for a patient in atrial fibrillation, with rapid ventricular rate but poor volume, gives a false impression since his actual heart rate may be much higher. It is useful to use the same symbols or colour system throughout the hospital to avoid confusion.

Calibration. The size of the ECG trace can be measured against a known standard. If the ECG machine is correctly calibrated an impulse of 1 mV causes a deflection of 10 mm. This is called standard calibration. (See Fig. 1.15.)

The same principles of paper speed and calibration are used in all types of monitoring equipment from electroencephalograms and electromyograms to pressure tracings. Calibration plays an enormously important part in all types of monitoring so that the value of a particular wave can be interpreted. It is set by the manufacturer in most pieces of equipment but may change as the instrument is exposed to various conditions such as temperature differences.

Base lines
In pressure monitoring equipment the base line may be set with reference to atmospheric pressure so, to compare the trace with set calibration, there must be a base line or zero line to represent atmospheric pressure. To achieve this a two-way tap is connected between the instrument and the line entering the patient. The tap is opened to atmospheric pressure. The infusion fluid drips out through the tap, and the pressure tracing on the screen becomes a horizontal straight line. Usually a control knob is available marked '0', baseline, shift or balance, to move the line up or down until it travels across the screen from a point on a scale marked as '0' or treated as the zero line. Sometimes a baseline continuously appears on the screen over which the pressure monitoring line must be placed exactly to achieve zero. The base line may represent 0 mm mercury or any amount that is convenient for a particular measurement.

Sometimes two, three or more readings appear on one screen, e.g. ECG, arterial pressure and venous pressure. Often the relation of one to another can be altered so it is important to decide which part of the screen is to be occupied by each. Separate calibration and points of reference are needed. There may be a scale marked at either side or different scales on one side. On older monitors, if two or more pressure traces appear on one screen it is useful to tape a graduated scale on either side for ease of reading it. This may be necessary when using versatile monitors on which different information can be displayed. The whole picture can become very confusing especially if one trace interferes with another. Different colours and separate digital displays clarify the readings considerably. Special care is needed if more than one patient's trace is displayed on the same screen.

Before taking any measurement or recording a trace it is important to check the base line and reset it if necessary, so that a point of reference is available. On some machines it rarely changes unless there is a fault. If it has to be altered every time a reading is taken it wastes a lot of nursing time so, if used often, more modern equipment might prove to be more reliable, and less time-consuming.

Other instruments, such as those used for measuring venous pressure, are subject to variables which make it necessary to check the base line immediately before every reading. A patient's position may change so equipment used for measuring central venous pressure is equipped with an arm fitted with a spirit level to line it up with a point of reference on the patient's body (see Chapter 6).

When recording some data on patient measurements it is important to demonstrate the calibration size used, particularly if a choice is available, e.g. the sensitivity of an ECG machine can be halved so that the trace fits on the paper, or doubled so that a small trace can be seen more clearly. This information can be written on the paper but conventionally, and more conveniently, the marker button is used to calibrate at the beginning of the trace or whenever the size of the trace is changed.

Electrical axis
The electrical axes of the heart are referred to the horizontal and frontal planes of the body. It describes the direction of the main flow of current in the heart. Unless qualified it refers to the QRS complex and the ventricles. The position of the heart and therefore the direction of the flow of electricity may be altered by bodily factors, e.g. during pregnancy or in obesity the heart may be lifted by the diaphragm to lie more horizontally. If a person has a tall, lean build the heart may lie more vertically (Fig. 1.17).

Willem Einthoven (1860–1927) discovered a system of studying electrical events in the heart by using a surface electrode attached to each limb and using the right foot, in contact with

Fig. 1.17. The average direction of flow of the electricity which produces the QRS complex (electrical axis) may be altered from normal by variations in body build.

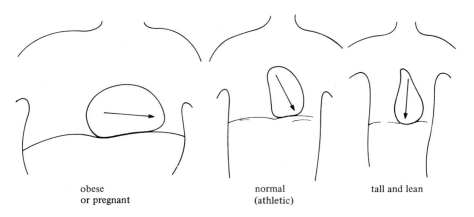

obese
or pregnant

normal
(athletic)

tall and lean

the floor, for earthing or 'grounding' the person. He measured the potential (i.e. the difference in voltage) in relation to the earth, which has a voltage of zero, between pairs of electrodes attached to the limbs (Fig. 1.18).

By comparing the flow of current in relation to the positive and negative poles the electrical axis can be discovered. The Einthoven triangle, which demonstrates the relationship of one pair of electrodes to another, is shown in Fig. 1.19. Leads I, II and III are bipolar (i.e. with two poles). Leads aVR, aVL and aVF are unipolar (i.e. single pole).

For ease of studying the electrical axis in the frontal plane

Fig. 1.18. Electrode link-up for limb bipolar and unipolar leads. The arrow on each figure points towards the direction from which the electrical current is viewed. The positive and negative electrodes in relation to the heart are shown for each lead. R, right side.

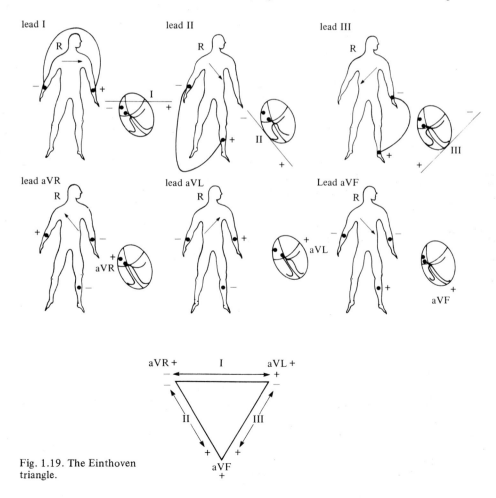

Fig. 1.19. The Einthoven triangle.

the Einthoven triangle may be redrawn as a six pointed star. (Fig. 1.20.)

To discover the frontal plane electrical axis of the heart look at the limb leads of a 12 lead ECG. Study the ECG in Fig. 1.21. Choose two leads which lie at 90° to each other for greater accuracy of drawing and convenience, e.g. lead I and lead aVF. Draw two lines at 90° to one another. The horizontal line represents lead I and the vertical line is lead aVF (Fig. 1.22a).

Look first at lead I. Count the number of small squares above the isoelectric line (7) and the number below the isoelectric line (1). Subtract them: the answer will be either a minus or a plus number, depending whether there are more below or above the line. In this case it is a plus number (6).

Now look at lead aVF. Count the squares above and below the isoelectric line and find the difference: plus or minus (−2).

Plot the results on the axes drawn; first lead I. As the answer is plus mark off the number along the right half from the central

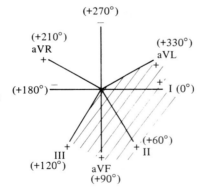

Fig. 1.20. The Einthoven triangle with the lead axes redrawn for ease of working out the electrical QRS axes of individual patients. The shaded areas represent limits of normal axis.

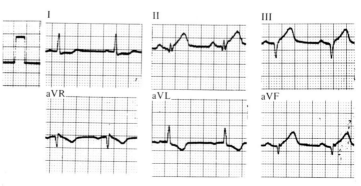

Fig. 1.21. A 12 lead ECG.

point, i.e. the positive end, using any convenient scale. Next, using the same scale, mark off the number on the vertical line, again being careful to check whether the result is plus or minus (Fig. 1.22b).

Now drop a perpendicular from the end mark on each line. Draw a line drom the centre point to the place where they cross. This line points in the direction of the mean vector of the QRS complex. In this case it is +340° i.e. within normal limits (Fig. 1.22c).

Normal limits are usually in the left inferior quadrant, but extend from plus 330° to plus 120° moving clockwise. This is a fairly accurate method. The use of a protractor is helpful if free-hand drawing is inaccurate.

Hypertrophy of the right or left ventricle may cause a shift of axis to right or left respectively.

Conduction disturbances to either anterior or posterior parts of the left bundle branch are a more frequent cause of a swing in

Fig. 1.22.

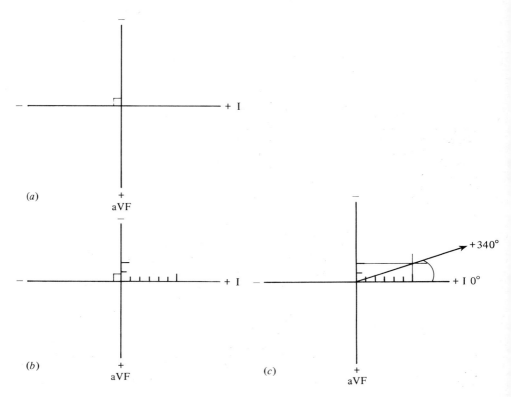

electrical axis. The change of axis is often a diagnostic feature (Fig. 1.23).

Study the ECG shown and try to work out the axis using the method described (Fig. 1.24; answer on p. 20).

Various rhythms are mentioned in this book so a short summary may be helpful.

Normal sinus rhythm (SR). (See Fig. 1.8.) Arises from the sino-atrial node, passes through the atrio-ventricular node taking no longer than 0.2 s before stimulating the ventricles. Entire depolarization lasts less than 0.12 s. It is a regular rhythm at a rate between 60 and 100 beats/min.

Sinus bradycardia. Arises from the S-A node at a rate less than 60 beats/min.

Sinus tachycardia. Arises from the S-A node at a rate greater than 100 beats/min in an adult.

Atrial tachycardia. (Fig. 1.25.) Arises from a fixed focus anywhere in the atria apart from the S-A node and discharges at a rapid rate (approximately 200 beats/min). The A-V node cannot conduct at more than about 180 beats/min and usually blocks some of the conduction so that the ventricles contract at a slower rate, often with a regular rhythm.

Atrial fibrillation. (Fig. 1.26.) Numerous foci in the atria discharge to produce rapid chaotic depolarization. The A-V node blocks most of the electricity and the ventricles are stimulated irregularly.

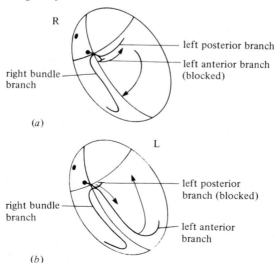

Fig. 1.23. Conduction defects are a more frequent cause of extreme axis deviation. (*a*) The main flow of electricity surges to the right, so there is right axis deviation; (*b*) the surge is to the left and upwards, resulting in left axis deviation.

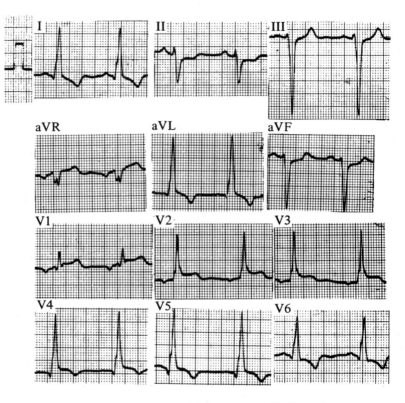

Fig. 1.24.

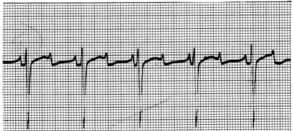

Fig. 1.25. A short strip of atrial tachycardia with an atrial rate of 136 beats/min. There is a 2:1 A-V block during tachycardia and the ventricular rate is 68 beats/min.

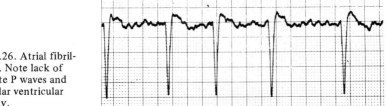

Fig. 1.26. Atrial fibrillation. Note lack of definite P waves and irregular ventricular activity.

Atrial flutter. (See Fig. 1.6.) Conduction from an ectopic focus spreads across the atria from one wall to another at a rapid rate (250–350 beats/min). A typical saw-tooth pattern is produced and is well seen in leads from the left leg (II, III and aVF) with usually regular ventricular stimulation, the A-V node causing an even block, i.e. 2:1, 4:1, 8:1, etc.

Junctional rhythm. (Fig. 1.27.) Arises from the atrio-ventricular node or nearby Bundle of His and stimulates the ventricles to conduct normally. Junctional bradycardia (less than 60 beats/ min) or junctional tachycardia (more than 100 beats/min) may occur. A P wave may be present immediately before or after the QRS and is inverted in II, III and aVF. This is caused by retrograde conduction.

First degree heart block (1°HB). The P-R interval is greater than 0.2 s implying delay in conduction between the S-A node and the ventricular muscle.

Second degree heart block (2°HB) (Fig. 1.28). There are several types. Heart block of 2:1 implies that every other sinus beat fails to stimulate the ventricles so there are two P waves to every QRS.

Complete heart block (CHB) (Fig. 1.29). The S-A node excites

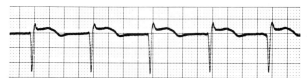

Fig. 1.27. Junctional rhythm.

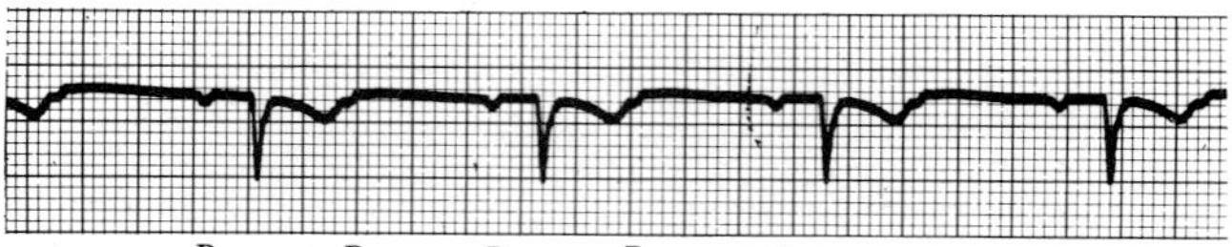

Fig. 1.28. 2:1 heart block – a second degree heart block.

Fig. 1.29. Complete heart block.

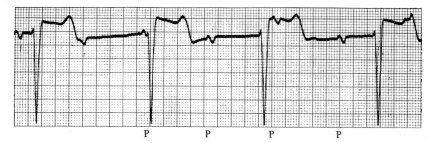

the atria at a regular normal rate but there is no consequent stimulation of the ventricles. Instead the ventricles contract at their own regular rate (escape rhythm), slower than the atria. The higher the focus is situated in the ventricles the faster the rate and the narrower the complex. A junctional rhythm is usual with block at the A-V node.

Ventricular rhythm. This may occur at any rate. Medium rate rhythm arising from a ventricular focus is often termed idioventricular rhythm (Fig. 1.30). Ventricular bradycardia is usually termed 'slow ventricular rhythm' and is the usual escape rhythm in complete block in the bundle branches (Fig. 1.31). Ventricular tachycardia arises from one focus in the ventricle although it may move and give varying patterns (Fig. 1.32). Regular dissociated P waves may be seen especially if the rate is slow. Ventricular tachycardia is a dangerous rhythm which may predispose to cardiac arrest with ventricular fibrillation.

Ventricular fibrillation. This refers to rapid chaotic depolarization which fails to produce an organized contraction of the ven-

Fig. 1.30. Idioventricular rhythm. Note: a P wave appears before each QRS complex but it is unrelated. The PR interval is short at the first beat and becomes progressively longer.

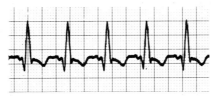

Fig. 1.31. Slow ventricular rhythm.

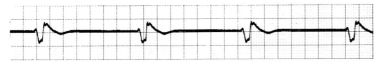

Fig. 1.32. A burst of ventricular tachycardia interrupts sinus rhythm.

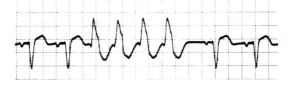

Fig. 1.33. Total atrioventricular block — P waves only are present.

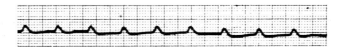

tricles which are unable to pump the blood so there is cardiac arrest (see Fig. 1.2 and Fig. 4.2).

Asystole. This is total absence of electrical events in the heart. It is another form of cardiac arrest and is usually seen as a straight line on the cardioscope.

CHB with failure of ventricular escape. (Fig. 1.33.) The atrial activity continues but the atrio-ventricular node and/or Bundle or His fail to conduct the electricity to the ventricles so there is no ventricular activity and no cardiac output.

The last three events mentioned, ventricular fibrillation, asystole and total atrio-ventricular block, all constitute *ventricular standstill* i.e. *no cardiac output* — an emergency condition requiring immediate action.

Further Reading

For further study of cardiac dysrhythmias there are many excellent books to be recommended, including:

Electrocardiograms — a systemic method of reading them.
     Michael L. Armstrong. Bristol; John Wright (1965).

The Heart. Frank H. Netter. The Ciba Collection of Medical Illustrations, vol. 5, ed. Frank Yorkman. New York; Ciba (1969).
     The Ciba Collection covers a particularly wide field and is beautifully illustrated. It could be useful with reference to many subjects mentioned briefly in this book.

Electrocardiography. Leo Schamroth. Oxford; Blackwell (1977).

Electrocardiography. John Hamer. London; Pitman Medical (1978).

An Atlas of Cardiology, Electrocardiograms and Chest X-rays.
     Neville Conway. London; Wolfe Medical (1977).

Electrocardiography. S.G. Owen. Boston; Little, Brown (1966).

Practical Electrocardiography. H.J.L. Marriot. Baltimore; Williams & Wilkins (1954).

Ans: +325° i.e. there is left axis deviation.

2. The electrocardiogram

By studying the variations from normal in the electrical patterns produced by the heart it is possible to diagnose fairly accurately the presence, site, size and age of a myocardial infarction. Myocardial infarction implies an area of heart muscle which has died as a result of complete lack of blood supply caused by blockage in a coronary artery, usually by atheroma, or sometimes by the interruption of blood flow by spasm in the coronary arteries. Ischaemia (lack of blood and therefore oxygen), hypertrophy (enlargement of cardiac muscle), pericardial effusion (fluid between the parietal and visceral layers of the pericardium) and dextrocardia (the heart and great vessels are twisted to lie in the intrathoracic cavity on the right side), can be demonstrated. The ECG is helpful in diagnosing the site from which dysrhythmias arise.

A complete picture is necessary for diagnostic purposes, demonstrating the electrical activity from various directions, basically anterior, inferior and lateral. Electricity from the posterior wall of the myocardium may be detected by electrodes applied across the patient's back, but the distance between the electrode and the heart is greater and therefore reduces the sensitivity. Also it is obviously inconvenient and may be impossible if the patient is collapsed. However, activation of the posterior wall can usually be detected in an anterior lead as a negative deflection since the current direction is away from the positive electrode. If this current is missing and replaced by an unusually large positive current, R wave, the presence of a posterior infarct can be deduced.

The standard 12 lead ECG records the activity from twelve different angles using an electrode attached to each limb and an electrode moved across the left anterior chest wall. The resultant record is termed an electrocardiogram.

Normally the limb electrodes consist of metal plates held in place by an adjustable rubber strap. For emergency use a clip-on electrode is available which looks like a large clothes peg. A suction device is provided for the chest wall, called an exploring electrode. Several types are available.

Study the diagrams of the Einthoven triangle (see Figs. 1.19 and 1.20). Standard limb leads I, II and III (see Fig. 1.18) are produced by moving a switch provided on the ECG machine, which connects appropriate pairs of electrodes, making one end positive and the other negative. Leads aVR, aVL and aVF are also automatically connected for correct recording. The resultant wave forms are amplified to be seen on the ECG paper.

Siting the chest electrodes is a little more difficult and should be positioned in the order given below (Fig. 2.1).

V1 Locate the sternum. Feel the ribs along the right sternal margin to find the fourth intercostal space.
V2 On left of sternal margin, opposite V1.
V4 Feel for the fifth intercostal space in the mid-clavicular line, usually just beneath the nipple.
V3 Intermediate between V2 and V4.
V6 Fifth intercostal space (remembering that the ribs curve upwards) in the mid-axillary line.
V5 Between V4 and V6.

Other chest (precordial) lead sites may be used to record more information. If the heart lies abnormally high or low in the thorax a position 5 cm above the usual sites are used and labelled E V1, E V2, etc., or 5 cm below and labelled L V1, L V2, etc. These are rarely used as there is little information on the normal range of patterns at these sites.

Recording a twelve lead ECG
To achieve a clear trace with minimal disturbance to the patient and least trouble to the technician, a few points should be considered.

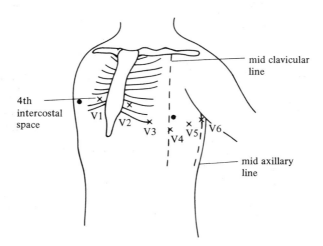

Fig. 2.1. Sites of electrodes for recording a 12 lead electrocardiogram.

The machine

Ensure all equipment is ready (Fig. 2.2):

4 metal electrodes ⎫
4 rubber straps   ⎬ ensure they are free of dried jelly and
1 chest electrode   ⎭ signs of corrosion
Electrode jelly
Spatula
Tissues
Pen
ECG paper
Skin marker if the ECG is first of a series

Electrode jelly

With many types of electrical apparatus a conducting medium is necessary to pick up clear signals from the body. It helps to transmit an electrical event quickly and clearly to an electrode attached to the body. If an electrode is inserted into the body, using a needle, no extra conducting medium is needed.

Some electrodes are used dry, especially with emergency equipment, but the trace achieved is often sub-standard. Various

Fig. 2.2. Portable battery or mains operated ECG machine with equipment.

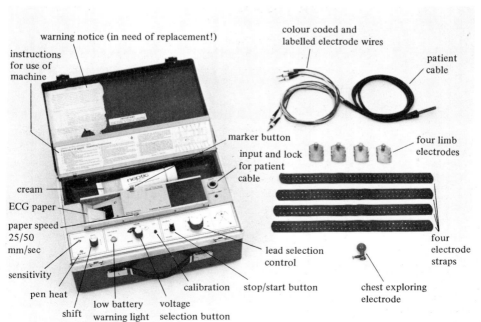

warning notice (in need of replacement!)

colour coded and labelled electrode wires

instructions for use of machine

patient cable

marker button

input and lock for patient cable

four limb electrodes

cream

ECG paper

paper speed 25/50 mm/sec

lead selection control

four electrode straps

sensitivity

pen heat

calibration   stop/start button

chest exploring electrode

shift   low battery   voltage
         warning light selection button

fluids can be used as a conducting medium, including saliva or even toothpaste, but many specially developed solutions are now used with excellent results. The recipe is basically the same with variations in the amount of electrolyte in a more or less jelly-like consistency. Included are glycerol monostearate, alcohol, sodium chloride, sodium bicarbonate, perfume and water with various other additions. Most produce no skin irritation but some, with higher sodium concentration, can cause redness. Thick conducting paste used for recording ECGs can be very abrasive and should be thoroughly washed off after use. It is not suitable for long-term monitoring.

Conducting jellies or creams are produced by many different firms, each claiming superior properties for them.

Lighting
Be sure the trace can be seen clearly by the technician.

Position of the machine
Place it on the patient's left side for ease of access to chest electrode, and face him. Switch on at the mains and the 'on' button to allow it to warm up, and ensure it works.

The patient
Explain in simple terms; help him to feel relaxed, and ensure he is warm as shivering causes interference from muscular tremor.

Position of the patient
The patient should lie flat on his back or semi-recumbent so that gravity helps the chest electrodes to remain *in situ*. Feet should not touch the end of the bed as tension in leg muscles produces a spiky trace. If he is very ill and should not move, remove the foot of the bed, or move his feet to either side. Head, arms and legs should lie in a relaxed manner. Use a pillow to support limbs held awkwardly because of intravenous lines or other attachments.

Application of electrodes
Place the limb electrodes where there is little hair and least amount of muscle to cause interference from tension, i.e. inner flat surface of wrists and ankles. Using a spatula, rub a small amount of jelly gently into the skin to abrade it slightly, improving electrode contact. Hold the four metal electrodes in place using light tension on the rubber straps. Attach the patient cable,

ensuring that each line, labelled on the end or at the junction
box, is secured to the correct limb. Colour code systems for the
limb leads differ, so do not rely on them until the machine
becomes very familiar. Wires should lie freely causing no tension
which produces interference and eventually weakens the cable.

Labelling
Before starting, at least write the patient's name, the date and
time. A note of the time is essential in a Coronary Care Unit
where events happen in quick succession, leading to serial ECG
records, all with the same date.

Calibration
This is often called sensitivity. The ECG is recorded at a standard
size for ease of comparison of a series of traces from individual
patients or a group. The height of the complexes increase if the
muscle enlarges, producing a greater voltage, e.g. large P waves
demonstrate atrial hypertrophy; large R waves may indicate
ventricular hypertrophy. A uniformly small trace may indicate a
very obese person, or pericardial effusion as fluid between muscle
and electrode interferes with conduction of electricity. Conventionally a square mark measuring 10 mm is used which represents 1 mV and is usually marked as ×1 on the machine (see
Chapter 1). If, in any single lead, the trace cannot be discerned
the sensitivity can be doubled by selecting the ×2 button. A
trace that will not fit on the squared part of the paper is halved
by selecting the ×½ button. It is only changed if really necessary
and it is important to label the trace accordingly, e.g. V 2 (½).
aVF (2), or preferably calibrate each individual lead.

Speed
Normal recording speed is 25 mm/s. As this is standard, no note
is usually made on the trace. If the speed is doubled to 50 mm/s,
to stretch out separate components to view more fully, it should
be stated (Fig. 1.16).

Everything is now ready to record the ECG. Calibrate at the
beginning. Move the selection switch to lead 1. On most machines
the stylus will move vertically from a central point with each
heart beat. Move the stylus using the position button so the trace
is drawn approximately across the middle of the paper. Timing
the movement of the stylus, run the machine to write out three
complete complexes. With practice this saves time and paper,

although some doctors may prefer more beats. If the rhythm is irregular, e.g. atrial fibrillation (see Fig. 1.26), about three seconds in each lead is advisable. Ensure the trace is free of tremor. If interference is present seek the cause (see 'Problems Page' at the end of this chapter). Sometimes a patient is so tense that muscular tremor persists, then record the chest leads first, which are less affected by tension, giving the patient more time to relax (Fig. 2.3). If the trace is clean, progress through the limb leads in order, moving the position of the stylus when necessary.

Mark the name of the lead above the trace as soon as it is recorded remembering to note calibration changes. Avoid writing on the squared paper so the label does not interfere with the trace when it is mounted. Some machines have a marker button which can be pressed as each lead is recorded and others mark them automatically.

In Lead II and aVF a non-pathological Q wave often appears which can be confusing when diagnosing presence of myocardial infarction, usually diagnosed from the presence of large Q waves. To minimize confusion ask the patient to take a deep breath while recording a second strip. Both recorded strips are often mounted and marked appropriately (IIR and aVFR).

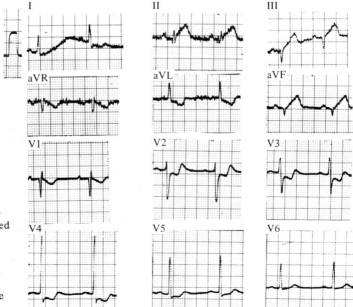

Fig. 2.3. 12 lead ECG shows somatic tremor in the limb leads caused by tensed muscles. If the patient cannot immediately relax record the chest leads first where it can be seen that there is little interference.

Now the chest leads. Attach the exploring electrode to the chest wire. Using a spatula to apply jelly, place a small blob on each site. Do not allow the blobs to join up. Too much jelly causes the electrode to slide out of position and it will be sucked inside the electrode. Place the electrode over V1 and progress to V6, stopping the motion of the stylus by moving the selector switch to a neutral position before the electrode is moved each time. If left in a recording position the rapid bizarre movement of the stylus will, in time, weaken the mechanism and it causes noise disturbing to the patient. To record V6 accurately the patient may need to move his arm away from the side. A wavy baseline is usually caused by respiratory movement. Ask the patient to breathe in, out and to hold his breath briefly after having exhaled. The chest is in a relaxed state so three complexes can be recorded with a straight base line. Encourage a patient in respiratory distress to breathe more shallowly while recording chest leads to lessen interference. Timing is all-important to achieve a good trace on a ventilated patient. Record before the inspiratory phase while the chest is still.

A strip of about ten seconds continuous beats completes the recording. This demonstrates the rate and rhythm and should include any irregularities. A longer strip is helpful if the irregu-larities are complex. The rhythm is often recorded in lead II but, if the monitoring lead on the cardioscope is different, e.g. V1, use this in preference. Use lead II or aVF if the atrial activity is of special interest or if P waves are indiscernable in lead V1. Lead V1 demonstrates ventricular dysrhythmias more accurately. The rhythm strip is usually recorded at the end of the ECG but, for speed, it could be taken during the ECG while the particular lead is connected. If any dysrhythmia arises during a recording, con-tinue to record the lead connected at the time until the dys-rhythmia stops or is obviously going to continue for some time.

Before removing the electrodes double check all points. If inexperienced ask a practiced colleague to inspect the trace before disconnecting the leads.

If the patient is co-operative the procedure should be com-pleted within five minutes. Wipe the jelly from the patient using a tissue, but a patient with a particularly hairy chest may need a wash to remove it properly. If the ECG is first of a series mark the site of chest electrodes with a skin pencil. This ensures uni-formity for comparisons, speed in emergencies and greater accu-racy as more care will be taken during the initial ECG.

Care of the equipment

Between patients wipe jelly off the electrodes, squeezing it from inside the chest electrode. When finished leave the machine clean and ready for instant use.

Wash the metal plates, chest electrode and rubber straps. Pay special care to the chest electrode, using a brush in the crevices. When dry, reconnect straps to electrodes; a dusting of powder makes them more pleasant to handle. Wipe jelly from the ends of the patient cable and wash them regularly. Replace top of the tube of jelly to prevent it drying out. Replenish stocks of paper, spatulae, tissues and jelly.

Some difficulties

Anatomical problems and attachments sometimes complicate ECG recording.

Obese patients. Ribs may not be felt so use the clavicle, nipple and mid-axillary lines as markers.

Pendulous breasts. The electrode should be against the rib cage so ask a colleague or the patient to support the breast while recording V4 and V5. If placed over the breast they may be inaccurate and could diminish the trace amplitude.

Amputee. Treat the most distal part of the stump as ankle or wrist and place the electrode on the inside surface. If there is no stump place it on the part of the body nearest the amputation site, using a plaster to keep the electrode in place.

Dextrocardia. This is a rare condition where the heart occupies the right side of the chest with its apex pointing towards the right foot. To take an accurate ECG comparable with a normal ECG connect the leads so the right arm lead is on the left arm, and vice versa. Mark the chest differently; place V2 in the normal place and record first, then V1 in its normal site. Now progress across the right chest wall to the mid-axillary line, marking the ECG paper as V2, V1, V3R, V4R, V5R, V6R.

Attachments, e.g. intravenous or arterial lines, plaster casts, clothing. If the area is merely covered by bandage (e.g. holding a splint) remove it for the duration of the recording. Perhaps it can be replaced differently for ease of access. Whenever possible the patient should have his chest bared for the ECG, so wearing a vest under pyjamas is to be discouraged.

Always place the electrode as near the usual site as possible. If one limb electrode has to be placed on the upper arm leave the other as usual. Never place the electrodes over stockings as, apart

from being a messy practice, there is likely to be excessive interference due to poor contact.

Other techniques
Further electrode sites are available for demonstration purposes.
These include extending chest leads to record at V7, V8 and V9,
giving a direct posterior view. An oesophageal electrode can be
swallowed to lie close to the atria, giving an enlarged view of atrial
action, but this has been largely superseded by an intracardiac
electrode, as for pacing.
Pericardial tap. To assist a doctor to aspirate a pericardial effusion,
the chest wire may be connected to the aspirating needle using a
wire attached by sterile crocodile clips. A normal chest lead trace
is recorded while the needle tip lies in the pericardial sac, but if
it touches the myocardium the ST segment rises warning the
doctor.
Pacing. While inserting a temporary pacemaker wire, the V lead
of the machine can be attached to the end of the pacing electrode, thus recording cardiac activity as the wire passes through
the right atrium into the ventricle. It may be a helpful guide to
the doctor during the procedure if no X-ray equipment is available, but cannot be regarded as an ideal method.

Mounting an ECG
There are many different methods of preparing the ECG for
patients' records. Each lead may be cut out and stuck on paper,
or a cardboard envelope with plastic windows is available from
some manufacturers, but it is expensive and cumbersome. Plastic
sleeves are available which have a slot at the top for the ECG
request card with details of the patient and a space for each sec-
tion of the 12 lead ECG which fits in without trimming, so time
is not wasted in cutting or glueing. The ECG is protected so the
original copy is preserved without the added expense of photo-
copying. Ensure original ECGs mounted in this way are not left
in direct sunlight or stored in a warm atmosphere, or the plastic
will act like a greenhouse and heat the 'thermosensitive' paper so
black patches will develop.
    Here are the main points when mounting the ECG: it must be
clearly labelled with the patient's full name, the date, time if
noted, and each lead clearly marked. A calibration mark should
precede the recording and any lead recalibrated should demonstrate the different size mark. Each complex should be complete.

Choose a uniform number of complexes throughout the ECG, e.g. two or three. However, if dysrhythmias occur these must be included (and not omitted to neaten it!). If the top and bottom are trimmed off, use a system to ensure each piece is cut out and stuck the right way up. Remember that most ECGs are drawn on heat-sensitized paper which reacts to body temperature and will scratch easily so handle with care.

Other types of ECG machine

Multichannel recorders

These are useful machines for diagnosing rhythm disturbances, as three or four leads are recorded simultaneously. This is achieved by attaching and connecting the limb leads as usual, then six separate chest electrodes are provided which each consist of a metal disc held in place by suction exerted along a tube by a large rubber bulb. Jelly often creeps up the tube, clogging it and preventing suction. Dried jelly around the hole in the metal disc also stops suction. The large, heavy rubber bulbs will drag the electrodes off the skin so they must be carefully placed to rest on the patient or bedclothes to help keep them in place. Each chest wire is colour coded and labelled. A colour chart stuck on the machine is helpful.

Calibration takes time as the size of the mark is reliant on how much the gain button is turned for each of the channels. If possible the machine should be left for instant use on $\times$ 1 mV calibration.

The position button usually needs moving for each set of recordings, to prevent crossing over and to keep the top and bottom lines on the paper. In a four-channel machine three groups of tracings are taken, for example:

I	II	III	V1
aVR	aVL	aVF	V2
V3	V4	V5	V6

Good positioning of the machine and patient are essential so the leads are not pulled or fall off. It sounds complicated, but with a co-operative patient, leads correctly attached, calibration and position chosen, the entire trace takes only half a minute to complete.

In some multichannel machines the ECG is drawn in ink which

is blotted by an absorbent roller. One ink bottle supplies the four pens and it is simple to remove the empty one and replace it. Occasionally the rate of ink flow needs adjusting. The blotter is not disposable: it consists of a cylindrical tube of porous material which is cleaned by using apparatus that allows a jet of tap water to enter one end of the hollow tube while the other end is closed off. The water passes through the absorbent material, cleaning off the ink. It dries out in about 24 hours, so a spare is necessary.

A multi-channel ECG machine is particularly useful for recording tachydysrhythmias, to help decide whether it is of supraventricular or ventricular origin. As leads I, II, and III are recorded simultaneously the change in axes can be studied from one beat to another. As II and V1 are recorded simultaneously they can be compared to pinpoint the P wave which may not be immediately evident on lead V1 (Fig. 2.4).

It is used also during stress tests when the heart rate is deliberately increased. Such factors as the QT interval can be more accurately measured.

Fig. 2.4. ECG taken with a multi-channel recorder. The ectopic activity is demonstrated from four directions simultaneously.

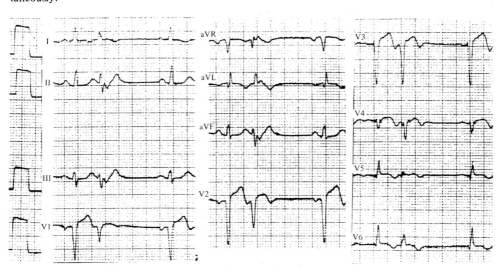

Holter monitors

Some people experience intermittent dizzy spells or syncopal attacks but when an ECG is recorded no abnormality appears. If the patient is attached to a cardioscope it may be several days before any symptoms occur.

In this instance a Holter monitoring device is invaluable in providing diagnostic evidence. Electrodes are placed on the patient's chest and are attached to a tape or cassette recorder which is light enough for the patient to carry easily at all times so that he can perform all his normal activities. The ECG is recorded continuously in one or two leads, typically lead II and lead V1 are chosen, or lead II if only one is used. Some recorders provide a button so the patient can mark the tape if he experiences symptoms, or the patient is asked to make a note of the time and type of symptom. The tape or cassette is fed through an analyser such that symptoms and cardiac rhythms can be related (Fig. 2.5).

Fig. 2.5. Rhythm strip from a patient with a history of syncopal episodes recorded by a Holter monitor. The long pauses caused by sinus arrest and the atrial ectopics are features of sick sinus syndrome.

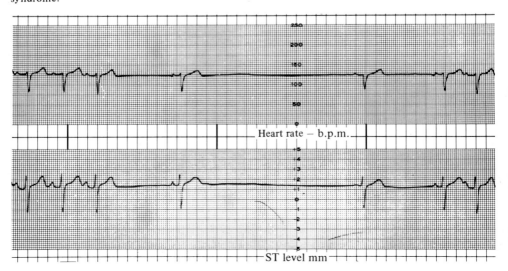

Problems page

Problem	Diagnosis	Remedy
Wavy base line (Fig. 2.6)	Excessive respiratory movement	Usually only apparent in chest leads. Before recording each chest lead ask the patient to hold his breath after exhaling. Record. As the chest is still and relaxed the base line should be straight
Thick line in chest leads only (Fig. 2.7)	Poor contact of chest electrode or wire	Wipe off excess jelly. Clean out inside of exploring electrode. Wash off dried or green jelly
Thick line in sets of leads	Poor contact of one limb lead, e.g. right arm lead affects leads I, II and aVR	Clean electrode, paying special care to hole in which wire is placed
Thick line in full ECG	(a) ECG paper wrongly threaded	(a) Re-thread paper
	(b) Earth lead interference	(b) Clean it or re-attach if disconnected
	(c) Mains interference (50 cycle/s fuzz)	(c) Disconnect any electrical appliances that are not vital, e.g. fan, electric thermometer

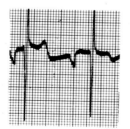

Fig. 2.6. Wavy baseline caused by deep breathing or poorly placed electrodes.

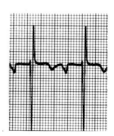

Fig. 2.7. Thick trace followed by improved recording as the earth electrode is connected.

	(d) Stylus heat too great	(d) Reduce heat by turning appropriate screw on machine, using insulated screw driver
Faint trace	Stylus heat insufficient	Increase heat as above
Spiky line (Fig. 1.14)	Muscular interference	Encourage patient to be still and relaxed. Ensure feet are not touching the bed at the bottom. Support limbs, head and back.
Spiky line (Fig. 2.8)	Electrical interference	Find the source and switch off the item if possible
Chest electrode falls off	Too much jelly on chest Patient is too upright	Wipe off excess jelly Allow patient to lie flatter
Puckered paper	Tension on paper is too great	Re-thread paper. Release tension with screwdriver
Bizarre, erratic movement in chest leads only	(a) Poor contact in chest electrode (b) Patient cable not properly plugged in	(a) Clean electrode and wire (b) Firmly re-attach patient cable to ECG machine

Fig. 2.8. Sinus rhythm followed by a spiky trace. This is not a dysrhythmia, although it may be picked up as such by a recording instrument: it is electrical interference.

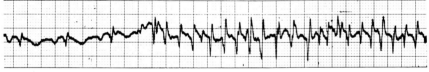

3. Monitoring with the aid of a cardioscope

Cardioscopes have been available for many years in hospital wards, the operating theatre, and are used while transporting patients and in special monitoring units. More recently cardioscopes have been usefully taken to the scene of an accident, or by specially equipped Coronary Ambulance to an office, factory or railway station.

Cardioscopes may be battery or mains operated, or both options may be provided on one machine. There are also models available that are operable from a car battery (Fig. 3.1).

Simple models display heart beats with a choice of two speeds — 25 mm/s (normal) or 50 mm/s. When the speed of the trace is set at normal the practised eye can tell the rate with fair accuracy. On a Coronary Care Unit changes in rate can occur rapidly and it is useful to see the information immediately displayed. Displays include a marker which swings across a numbered scale, or a line across the cardioscope which becomes longer or shorter as the rate changes. These are called analogue displays. A digital display of illuminated numbers is probably most easily seen from across the ward. Ensure that the rate is registered accurately. Small voltage beats, such as ventricular ectopics may be ignored by the machine. Conversely, if the amplitude control is too high every

Fig. 3.1. Mains or battery operated portable cardioscope with choice of two speeds, three calibration sizes, rate metre and choice of monitoring lead.

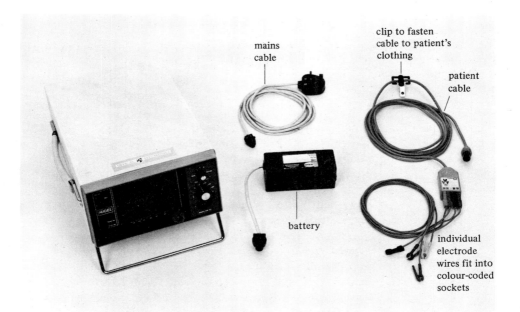

mains cable

clip to fasten cable to patient's clothing

patient cable

battery

individual electrode wires fit into colour-coded sockets

beat may be counted twice as the T wave will also trigger the recorder. This check is particularly important if an alarm system is incorporated which triggers if the rate falls below or rises above a pre-set limit. The electrical stimulus (artefact) discharged by a pacemaker can be counted as a heart beat even if no ventricular depolarization occurs (see Chapter 5). Electrical interference producing a spiky trace may be counted as a tachycardia (Fig. 2.8).

The height of the trace may be altered by turning a control knob marked 'gain', 'amplitude', 'size' or 'sensitivity', or it may be marked with a shape implying increase or decrease. The size of the trace should not be increased so far that it is distorted or causes a flattening of the top or bottom of the complex. Some machines incorporate a numbered wheel next to a light source. When the wheel is turned to its lowest position a small trace is seen. The small R waves are not detected so the light does not flash. The wheel is turned, increasing the amplitude, until the light flashes on every R wave. Increase it a little more to allow the patient changes of position, which may decrease the amplitude. This method minimizes the risk of large T waves being counted as R waves which would give a double rate reading.

As the trace moves across the screen from left to right the preceding beats gradually fade away, but slowly enough to allow comparisons of a few beats so that trends can be studied. Other systems display cardiac rhythm which moves in a continuous band from left to right or right to left. Some nurses find the first system easier to watch but it is a matter of preference.

Some machines display the rhythm on two lines so that one line can be stopped by pressing a 'freeze' button, for more careful study.

Individual bedside cardioscopes may be connected to a central console at the desk where all patients' heart beats can be seen simultaneously. There may be several lines displayed, up to ten at times, but it is possible, with practice, to note the rhythm disturbances in any one patient as the normal pattern for that patient is interrupted. It is impractical to ask any one person to study the main console to report dysrhythmias for 15 minutes or even less. Studies have shown that many rhythm disturbances are still missed. General trends can be observed by experienced staff glancing at the main console from time to time. Often they are unaware of looking at the console until an abnormal event occurs which is noted. A system may be evolved where the console is studied for five minutes continuously every hour; the type and number of ectopic beats can be noted and recorded on the patient's chart. Trends can be seen which may decide the nurse to observe a particular patient more closely.

A write-out device may be incorporated which can be used to print out any patient's rhythm for as long as a button is pressed or for a short strip. The type which allows any length of rhythm strip is preferable as it saves paper if only a few beats are needed, and allows changes of rhythm to be written out without interruption. An alarm system may be connected to the write-out machine. Immediately an alarm signal occurs it automatically writes out the rhythm, which can be studied later. There is usually a timed delay of about five to seven seconds, by which time the dysrhythmia will be established. To find the cause of the disturbance it is useful to have a memory tape or cassette in the system. This records continuously on tape, which is wiped clean as new data is fed on to it. It stops automatically after a timed delay when an alarm signal occurs. At leisure it can be replayed, displaying approximately ten seconds of rhythm before the disturbance occurred, demonstrating the activity causing a change in rate. It continues to write-out the rhythm, the entire tape lasting between 30 and 60 seconds, depending on preference. This helps the doctor to decide what treatment should be given to prevent further similar problems. Memory tapes are not available on any current system. More modern systems do not store analogue ECG data on tape but record digital ECG information in digital memory stores. This information is continuously updated and may be retrieved as hard copy on ECG paper.

Tape units can be useful in writing out rhythms seen briefly on the cardioscope, which need further study. Tangible evidence is then available demonstrating the rhythm for diagnosis, discussion and teaching. When rhythm strips are recorded it is wise to mark it with the patient's name, the time and the date. Strips of particular interest are best mounted on paper and labelled immediately, especially when medication or other treatment is given.

As mentioned, the alarm system is activated by a change in rate beyond the pre-set limits set on a cardioscope monitoring an individual patient. Should the cardiac rhythm be disturbed without a change in rate this will not be noted using this system, e.g. normal sinus rhythm at a rate of 70 beats/min may change to junctional rhythm at a similar rate but with absent P waves, or a ventricular rhythm where the complexes are wide and the heart may be in jeopardy.

Analysers have been developed to note such parameters as width of QRS, and absence or excess of atrial activity. Many false alarms occur and a lot of subtle changes are missed which can be seen by the human eye. Although there is room for improved accuracy, these alarm systems play an important role in monitoring patients in high dependency areas where the nurses can rarely spend time in watching monitors continuously.

In hospital a doctor may request that a patient is monitored on a general ward. The equipment often comes from a different area and the nurse needs to know that it is complete and works before she sets it up on the patient. It comprises the monitor, mains cable or well-charged battery, patient cable to attach the electrodes to the monitor and correct electrodes to fit the cable. Many monitors have a light to show whether mains or battery is in use.

However simple or complicated the apparatus, the most important aspect of monitoring is the application of electrodes to give a clear trace, to maintain adherence, and their placement at appropriate sites. The doctor is often not available to watch the monitor for any length of time, so if a good trace is achieved at once and the senior nurses, at least, recognize normal rhythm for the patient and can distinguish interference from dysrhythmias, everyone will be more confident, especially the patient.

Types of electrodes

Pre-jelled electrodes
Pre-jelled disposable electrodes are an aid to good monitoring as they are quick to use and the amount of jelly provided is calculated to give optimum performance. There are several types available with different features. Prices vary, so economics may be a deciding factor when choosing electrodes for use in a particular ward or department; e.g. less expensive electrodes may be used for short-term monitoring during cardiac catheterization, while more expensive electrodes may be used for longer term monitoring in a Coronary Care Unit.

Types available include a pre-jelled plastic electrode with a central foam-rubber pad. It is a decent size (55 mm diameter) with good adherent qualities but tends to lift off when a patient perspires heavily. The longer it remains *in situ* the stickier it becomes if the skin is dry. When removing an electrode the natural tendency is to tear it off quickly as if it were elastoplast, but less abrasion is caused if it is slowly peeled off, using an ether solvent if necessary. The pad in which the central foam sits is fairly thick, which helps to cushion the metal electrode so that it is comfortable for thin people. This depth sometimes causes it to catch on bedclothes or against wires.

There is a micropore electrode with a central foam disc containing a low concentration silver chloride gel which is less irritant to the skin. It is claimed to adhere to heavily perspiring bodies. This is so, as long as it is used correctly with good skin preparation. Ensure that there are no creases in the paper when it is smoothed on to the skin. As it lies flat there is less danger of catching bedclothes or clothing, so there is less interference seen on the cardioscope. It covers a fairly large surface area being 73 mm in diameter.

Children's electrodes have a smaller sticky surface area but the gel contact is the same size as adult electrodes. The micropore variety are probably best for young sensitive skin. A sunny smiling face printed on them makes one brand popular with children. These can also be used on very small babies.

There are many others available which are all sizes, made of different materials, such as polystyrene, and in various shapes, including hearts and flowers. As more research is done, smaller and better electrodes will be produced.

Most pre-jelled electrodes stay firmly attached indefinitely and only need changing when they fall off, perhaps two weeks later. Few patients are sensitive to them, but if itching occurs, re-site the electrodes. The source of irritation may be the adherent area but more often it is the foam rubber or jelly in the centre. The jelly may have a high concentration of chloride causing small blisters which clear quickly when washed and exposed to air. Calamine lotion may prevent the patient scratching and breaking the blisters. If the problem is persistent, change to a different make of electrode, with a less concentrated medium.

Single dry electrodes
These are small disposable electrodes (30 mm diameter) attached to the patient cable by a push-in sleeve via a short wire. Ensure that there is a tight fit so that the cable does not slide out. The outer adherent disc is protected by paper. Jelly is required to conduct the electricity from the skin to the central electrode.

Any substance could be used as a medium, but non-irritant, water-soluble jelly is recommended. To apply the jelly, squeeze a small amount into the central indentation, then, using a spatula, scrape off any excess so that the jelly is flush with the top of the indentation. Peel off the protective paper disc and, having prepared the skin, apply the electrode firmly, pressing around the edge of the disc. If too much jelly is used the pressure will cause the jelly to creep under the sticky area, thus lifting the electrode. Too little jelly will impair conduction.

Non-pre-jelled electrodes are less expensive but take longer to put on and fall off more readily as they are smaller, less sticky and the jelly will move under the sticky area if pressure is applied. They usually need to be changed daily and are unsuitable for long-term monitoring.

Metal electrodes

The flat metal electrodes used for taking a 12 lead ECG may be used for temporary monitoring, such as during a cardiac arrest, before a proper monitoring system is set up. They should not be used for any length of time as the jelly will quickly dry out as it is not contained in an air-tight seal, thus producing a poor quality trace. Also it is uncomfortable for the patient and may cause circulatory impairment.

Mat for ECG monitoring

This is a disposable electrode system which consists of three metallic strips adhering to card which is placed dry under the left side of the patient's chest as he lies on his back. A clamp is attached to the card where it emerges at the shoulder, the other end being connected to a monitor. It is specifically useful during surgery and can be placed across the patient's back as he lies prone. It is X-ray translucent.

Patients nursed lying prone can be monitored using a foam pad with four electrodes embedded in it, which is connected to the monitor by a single cable.

Some electrodes cover a larger area on an X-ray than others and they are more or less opaque. Electrode opacity is not usually a problem unless it interferes with visualizing pacing wires (see Chapter 5) or with the diagnostic value of X-rays.

Site of the patient

In a monitoring unit all patients should be in sight of the desk where the monitor can easily be seen, or there should be a main console displaying all patients' rhythms. A patient in a general ward should be opposite the desk area where his monitor can be seen at a glance.

Before attaching the electrodes choose the site of the monitor if it is portable. The patient's locker is often used but it gives him less room for his possessions and he may turn the locker or stretch across it to reach a cupboard or shelf, endangering the monitor.

A separate table is better, preferably with a fiddle along the edge so there is less danger of the monitor falling off if the cable is tugged. A bedside table or heart table are both useful and can be placed so the monitor can be seen easily from the sister's desk and by nurses passing the bed, but is not in the patient's direct line of vision. If possible do not put the monitor where the patient can see it. A nearby window-sill above the patient is ideal.

In a monitoring unit the cardioscope is often mounted above and behind the patient on a purpose-built swivel shelf attached to the wall, so the monitor can be turned to the best viewing position. The cardioscope in the operating theatre is near the anaesthetist. It is often placed high up in a angiography theatre so that it is visible to all the technicians and doctors.

Application of electrodes

It is false economy not to apply the electrodes correctly even in an emergency. The whole procedure takes only a few seconds in practised hands when equipment is kept ready for use, so it makes good sense, especially in a busy monitoring unit, to have a special tray which is always replenished.

Have ready a tray containing: a razor which is ready for immediate use — either disposable or a cleaned razor with a new blade; a spatula; a spirit swab or spirit spray and tissue; a paper towel to collect shaved-off hairs; pre-jelled electrodes, or dry electrodes and jelly.

Switch on the monitor to warm it up and to ensure it works. Plug in the patient cable to be sure it fits the machine. Choose the electrode sites. All electrodes are placed on the trunk, not on the limbs as the muscles cause interference ('noise') when tense (see Fig. 2.3). Also there is less disturbing movement of the trunk, and the wires are less likely to be caught in clothing and bedding. Avoid areas where electrodes for a 12 lead ECG are placed or where paddles would be placed for defibrillation (see

Chapters 2 and 4). Do not place them on skin folds or where pendulous breasts will rest. Shave off any hairs over the chosen areas in a circle well clear of the edge of the electrode. Rub the area with a spirit-impregnated swab, cleaning off natural skin oils which may impede good conduction. By shaving and rubbing the skin it is slightly reddened, helping contact. Attached to some pre-jelled electrodes is an abrasive area, but be careful not to be too enthusiastic with this! If no shaving is needed the spatula can be used for abrading the skin. Allow the spirit to evaporate for a few seconds while attaching each electrode to the appropriate lead. Ensure the metal part of a snap-on clip makes contact with the metal knob on the electrode or there will be no conduction. Apply the pre-jelled electrode to the skin. Rub around the electrode with a finger, as heat will help it to adhere firmly. If the electrode has to be jelled, attach it to the correct lead before filling the indentation with jelly. Place it on the skin, using finger heat to assist it. Allow the patient cable to lie freely, causing no tension on the electrodes. If the patient is fairly active it is wise to attach the cable to his pyjamas — never to the bedclothes as they do not move with him. A safety-pin can be used but a specially manufactured cable clip is preferable. This is particularly useful when the patient stands out of bed as the clip will prevent the weight of the cable dragging the electrodes off. The cable should be long enough to allow uninhibited movement. A completely inactive patient poses no problems in keeping the electrodes attached for several days, but care must be taken while

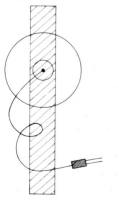

Fig. 3.2. A tension loop and plaster help electrodes to stay on longer.

turning him to prevent tension on the wires. Patients in a Coronary Care Unit or general ward are encouraged to move freely, so ensure they are not inhibited or annoyed by electrodes dropping off every time they turn over or cough. If it is obvious that further steps will be needed to keep electrodes *in situ*, take them before the patient becomes irritable at being disturbed, or the nurse turns off the alarm system. A tension loop in the wire is very effective (Fig. 3.2).

A few patients perspire very freely and although some manufacturers claim that the electrodes will adhere despite perspiration it is sometimes a difficult problem. Anti-perspirants used on the skin where the electrode sticks is often effective in severe cases. Micropore electrodes tend to remain attached. However, if these are unavailable, plaster may be the only answer.

Changing electrodes every day becomes very costly. Using plaster may be the only means of keeping electrodes on very active patients such as children or disturbed adults. Dermaclear and micropore plaster are useful as they adhere well, are porous, allow the skin to breathe and are less likely to cause irritation when used for long periods.

Pre-jelled electrodes are packed in sealed envelopes singly, in triple packs or loose in larger packets. All have an airtight seal over the central foam. However, once the outer package is broken air will dry out the jelly in time, despite this seal. Before applying pre-jelled electrodes, ensure the foam pad is damp, otherwise time will be lost in finding the dried electrode, giving poor contact. If only one electrode is needed, take it from a single pack rather than the triple packet to lessen the problem of the others in the pack drying out. The cost of a triple pack is usually the same as three singles, so it may be more economical to buy singles. It is not good practice to leave the electrodes attached to the cable ready for an emergency admission as it may be several hours or days before they are used and they may dry out. Shelf-life varies but usually they last at least a year if they are stored at a reasonable temperature, $25-45\,^\circ$C is recommended. The date is stamped clearly on the outer packing.

More information about electrodes is available in 'ECG Electrodes' K.G. Wiggins & S.J. Meldrum, *The British Journal of Clinical Equipment*, 2, 90–4 (1977) and *Techniques of Measurement – Electromedical*,

The patient cable may have attachments for three, four or five electrodes.

Five electrode system
This has a chest (V) lead and one lead for each limb. The monitor to which it is attached will usually provide a button for a choice of monitoring positions – I, II, III, aVR, aVL, aVF and V. If the chest lead is used it will pick up electricity only over the part of the chest where it is placed. Junior staff will find it easy to place labelled electrodes on the correct site and it may be an advantage to choose the lead in which to monitor by only turning a dial However, five electrodes can be cumbersome in nursing the patient. This system is used commonly on a general ward. The doctor may choose to view lead II by moving the selector switch on to lead II. Assuming normal sinus rhythm he should see a clear trace with a P wave, QRS complex and T wave. The monitor

uses the right arm lead (−ve), the left leg lead (+ve) and the right leg acts as the earth (Fig. 3.3).

Lead II usually shows atrial activity best, so it is the most suitable lead to use if the rhythm is atrial fibrillation, atrial flutter or atrial tachycardia.

Ventricular activity is often observed well using the chest lead. It is best placed centrally over the sternum or slightly to the right of the sternum where there is less muscle to cause interference. These areas avoid the sites of the V leads of the 12 lead ECG and sites for defibrillation. If the patient has ventricular dysrhythmias these are most easily interpreted using a chest lead.

The four-lead system
This allows choice of the equivalent of any limb lead (I to aVF) by placing the labelled electrode on the appropriate part of the trunk, i.e. right arm lead on the upper right area, etc. Use the dial on the cardioscope to choose the monitoring lead. Monitoring in an approximate V1 lead is possible by changing over the left leg and right arm wires. Move the dial to lead II.

The three-lead system
This has the advantages of economy of time and money, least trouble to the patient and the full range of leads to choose for monitoring, both limb and chest. To use this system to its best advantage one needs to learn which are the negative and positive poles of the pairs of leads on a 12 lead ECG (Chapter 2). The leads can be attached to carefully placed electrodes giving tracings

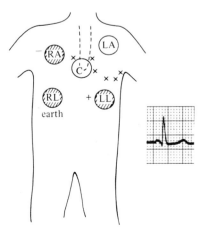

Fig. 3.3. Placement of five electrodes to monitor a modified lead II. The three shaded electrodes are those involved in recording lead II. P waves usually show clearly in this lead.

which, although not absolutely true, are accurate enough for a high standard of monitoring.

Most manufacturers label the three leads: right arm, left arm and right leg. This three-lead system is based on lead I of the 12 lead ECG and may be translated as:

right arm — negative pole
left arm — positive pole
right leg — earth

Colour code systems are employed on patient cables but it is useless if an electrode breaks and the correct colour is not immediately available and time may be wasted looking for it. Some systems state on the junction box to which limb the electrode belongs and a few state if it is negative, positive or earth.

In a Coronary Care Unit the ideal monitoring lead is V1 or modified chest lead I (MCL 1) with the positive electrode placed near the site of V1 of the 12 lead ECG. A negative electrode is required when using a monitor so place it on the opposite side of the heart but avoid the areas for defibrillation, V5, V6 and the axilla. The earth lead can be placed anywhere but it is sensible to put it on the side nearest the monitor, which is preferably on the patient's left side so the wires do not stretch across his chest. Placed in this position the earth electrodes can be used for monitoring in a different lead (Fig. 3.4).

It is the life-threatening dysrhythmias and their precursors that the Coronary Care nurse is most concerned about. Ventricular dysrhythmias, which may result in ventricular fibrillation, are observed well in lead V1.

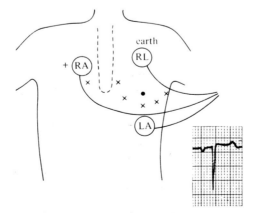

Fig. 3.4. Placement of three electrodes to monitor lead V1 or a modified chest lead I (MCL1).

Ventricular ectopics are seen clearly and it is often possible to say from which ventricle they arise (Chapter 1). This may be important if, for example, the patient has a pacing wire terminating in the right ventricle, and the monitor shows right ventricular ectopics. These may be attributable to the pacing wire so, by moving it (or the patient's position) the ectopics may stop rather than resorting immediately to medication (Fig. 3.5).

Bundle branch block, which may lead to trifascicular block and asystole is demonstrated most accurately using lead V1. The patterns seen on Figs. 1.11 and 1.12 are typical. Sinus rhythm with normal conduction and sinus rhythm with right bundle branch block look spectacularly different in lead V1.

If it is preferred to monitor in lead II change over the positive and negative leads to reverse the polarity. It is then similar to lead II. (Fig. 3.6).

If a patient develops sinus rhythm with right bundle branch block he can be monitored in lead aVF or lead III as the electrical axis of the heart will shift to right or left if conduction in one of the remaining bundles is impaired (see Chapter 1), and is often best seen in lead III (Fig. 3.7). On the cardioscope the pattern will alter markedly so a 12 lead ECG can be taken to confirm diagnosis.

Fig. 3.5. Sinus rhythm with right and left ventricular ectopic beats.

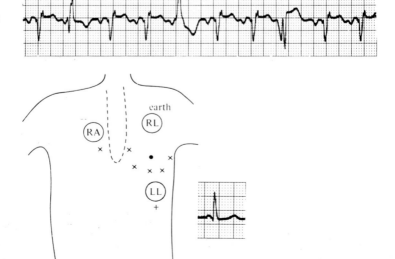

Fig. 3.6. Placement of three electrodes to monitor lead II.

When using three electrodes the patterns achieved are very similar to the 12 lead ECG. It should be noted if the monitoring lead is changed, and a rhythm strip run off. When monitoring in lead III, an ECG rhythm strip of lead III should be taken for comparison. If the lead III monitoring pattern changes, always confirm with a 12 lead ECG as it may only be that the patient has turned on to his side, causing his heart to lie nearer the recording electrode, thus increasing the size of the trace.

Having chosen the site and attached the electrodes, look at the monitor to ensure the trace is clear. When using a proper system for applying electrodes the trace should be good immediately.

Problems that may arise
Thick trace (Fig. 3.8). Check that the earth electrode is damp with jelly.

Scratch the skin a little under the earth electrode to aid contact. Scratch the skin under the other electrodes.

Check both ends of the wire attaching cable to electrode: are they properly connected? Are they clean?

Check the wire casing: is it broken?

Adjust the focus.

Other electrical equipment can cause interference. To find which is responsible, switch off each in turn, starting with the

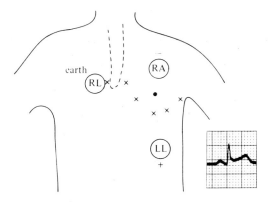

Fig. 3.7. Placement of three electrodes to monitor lead III.

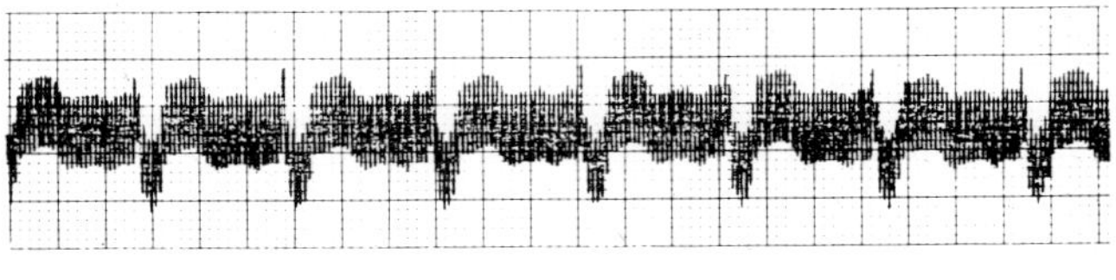

Fig. 3.8. Thick trace as chest electrode is gummed with jelly.

equipment nearest the patient. If the item is expendable leave it off, but if it is essential try plugging it into a socket further away.

If all these checks fail to achieve a good trace, change the earth lead wire, then the other electrode wires, then the electrodes, using careful skin preparation, then the whole patient cable. After that it must be a faulty monitor!

Straight line. The patient cable is not completely pushed into the socket on the cardioscope.

The positive or negative lead may not be making contact: are they properly attached? are they clean? A positive or negative electrode may be dry.

The gain control may be turned right down.

On a multi-channel recorder the wrong channel may be switched on.

The patient is asystolic.

Trace is too dim or too bright. The brightness control, usually at the rear of the machine, needs adjusting.

Blurred trace. The focus control needs adjusting.

These last two adjustments often need to be done with a screw-driver — not nurses' scissors. Always use an electrical screwdriver which has an insulated handle. An experienced Coronary Care nurse will usually carry one in her pocket.

Wavy line. Caused by patient's respirations, so replace the electrodes where there is less chest movement (see Fig. 2.6). By moving only the patient cable the problem may be solved.

Trace disappears from the screen intermittently. Indicates loss of contact. Check that the weight of the cable is not pulling at the electrodes. Adjust the cable slip (Fig. 3.9).

Are clothes or bedding lifting an electrode?

Are all points of contact clean?

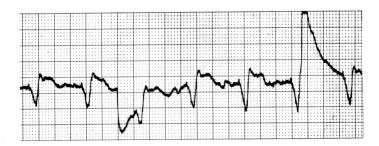

Fig. 3.9. Loss of electrode contact causes recording to slip intermittently.

Intermittent spikes. These are caused when other electrical items are switched on and off (Fig. 3.10).

Spiky trace. Usually caused by muscular tremor. Re-site electrodes in a less muscular area (see Fig. 1.14).

Shattered trace. This is usually caused by a broken electrode wire (Fig. 3.11).

Distorted image. The trace may be too large or too small.

Large loops on cardioscope whenever anyone walks near the monitor. This is caused by inadequate earthing of the cardioscope. An antistatic floor also helps to prevent pick-up. Care should be taken with the choice of floor covering.

Intermittent appearance of 'junctional' rhythm when using a write-out machine. A stiff stylus mechanism or build-up of matter on the stylus tip cause sluggish movement, so the P and T waves appear flat (Fig. 3.12). In this case the trace on the cardioscope will be different.

When the trace is satisfactory and the cable is firmly attached to the patient, set the alarm system if there is one to use. It is seldom possible to have one person watching a monitor constantly on a general ward or in a monitoring unit and it is unnecessary so long as the alarm system is reliable. A high and low alarm can be set to alert the nurse if the patient's rate slows below or speeds above a

Fig. 3.10. Intermittent spikes (↑) may appear on the monitor as other electrical apparatus is switched on and off.

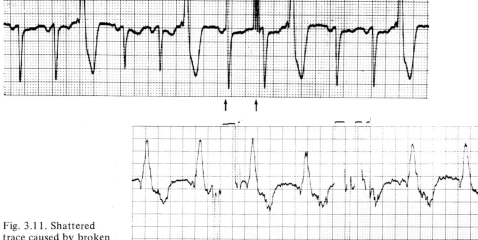

Fig. 3.11. Shattered trace caused by broken wire.

pre-set limit for more than a few seconds (seven seconds is reasonable). A low limit of 50 beats/min and upper limit of 100 beats/min is acceptable and can be adjusted as required. The signal may be either audible or visible, and is often both. Some alarms sound very distressing while others have a pleasant tone which is more acceptable to patients, visitors and staff.

Avoid unnecessary alarm signals which cause tension to all and may result in the alarm system being switched off on a particular patient. If it repeatedly alarms, find the cause and deal with it: do not just switch off the alarm. Some systems automatically write out a rhythm strip lasting a few seconds, so if false alarms occur, large amounts of paper can be wasted.

Re-positioning a patient for an X-ray, washing him or moving him to relieve pressure may cause interference, resulting in false alarms, so switch off the system temporarily. As someone is with the patient the monitor can be observed. When a patient sits out of bed on a commode, turn off the alarm system if there is a main console where the rhythm can be watched to prevent needless interruption of his privacy. Always remember to reset the alarm afterwards.

Other staff who treat patients should be taught to use the alarm system so that they are aware of its implications and can switch it off when there is a possibility that interference will cause a false alarm. Before the physiotherapist begins chest and limb exercises she should be encouraged to switch off the system, and to remember to reset it at the end of treatment.

When a cardiac arrest occurs, turn off any audible alarm signals as soon as it is convenient to prevent further distress to other patients. The resuscitation team can see the rhythm.

While inserting a pacemaker wire an experienced person watches the monitor constantly so the alarm can be switched off as no signal is needed (Chapter 5).

For emergency use a small cardioscope is available which is

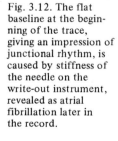

Fig. 3.12. The flat baseline at the beginning of the trace, giving an impression of junctional rhythm, is caused by stiffness of the needle on the write-out instrument, revealed as atrial fibrillation later in the record.

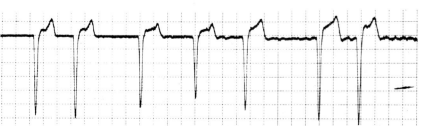

used without attaching electrodes to the patient. It is simply placed over the chest where three electrodes on the back of the machine make contact with the skin. No electrode cream is necessary but if there is poor contact any jelly can be used, or even saliva. One model has a 6 V battery with a life of about six months, or it can be run off the mains. If the monitor is needed for long periods, such as transferring a patient, it can be run from car batteries. Further attachments can be provided such as a tape unit to record the rhythm or spoken comments, and a cable for continuous monitoring with limb electrodes attached. A polaroid camera will photograph the rhythm for later interpretation. The model is suitable for use with children or adults as two sizes of interchangeable electrode plates are provided.

Before detaching a patient from a monitor turn off the alarm signals prior to removing the electrodes and turning off the mains supply. Some machines give an alarm signal if the mains current is disconnected. More sophisticated machines have a different alarm for loss of ECG when a lead falls off.

The conscious patient should be involved with the care of his monitoring equipment to give optimum performance, to preserve it in good condition and to achieve a constant high quality trace with fewest alarm signals. He should be discouraged from scratching the electrodes, causing 'ventricular fibrillation' on the monitor (Fig. 3.13), fiddling with the cable, causing 'ventricular tachycardia' (Fig. 3.14), or disconnecting the electrodes causing 'asystole'.

Fig. 3.13. Sinus rhythm with regular superimposed artefacts may look like ventricular fibrillation at a glance and may set off some automatic alarm systems.

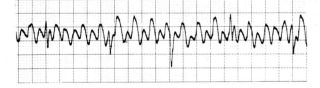

Fig. 3.14. Ventricular tachycardia? This is actually sinus rhythm at about 50 beats/min with a large artefact on top.

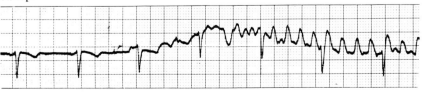

If an electrode falls off or a couple of wires become disconnected, do not assume that the patient or other untrained person has replaced them correctly. Encourage the patient to inform the nurse as an altered pattern may cause her to think his rhythm has changed.

Care is needed when dressing patients so that the cable and wires are untangled and project from the clothing in a convenient place for patient and nurse, with the least tension on electrodes. It is best to run the cable up over the head of the bed where it can be taped in position, leaving plenty of slack.

Even the least sick patient needs help while moving in and out of bed until he is thoroughly used to the length of the cable and where it is attached. It is easy to trip over long cables or to catch them around chair arms, or knobs on lockers.

Care of the patient attached to a cardioscope
This includes skin care, careful siting of electrodes and monitor, avoidance of pressure sores from wires and cable, cleaning and regular maintenance of the machine by qualified technicians. Psychological factors must also be considered.

Most patients accept a cardioscope as a modern aid to good medical care but others become anxious about its implications. Relatives tend to watch the cardioscope and patients will look at other patients' rhythms as well as their own if the monitor is in sight. The very act of turning to look at his monitor can cause interference to the pattern which may frighten him. Simple explanations will help, but the maxim 'a little knowledge is a dangerous thing' applies to both relatives and patients. It can be exasperating if a patient constantly points out 'dysrhythmias', but a gentle, matter-of-fact attitude which should come naturally to the Coronary Care nurse will allay fears and renew confidence.

Wherever a patient is attached to a cardioscope the staff caring for him should be competent to use the equipment or it can be worrying for the nurse and upsetting to the patient. If the doctor is the only person to look at the monitor twice a day and never at night he should perhaps only attach the patient to the machine for that length of time or take a 12 lead ECG.

If monitoring is to play a serious part in preventive medicine the equipment and staff must be adequate for the job, so specialized areas should be used to their full potential. A Coronary Care Unit is often misnamed as patients are admitted with all types of conditions requiring the use of a cardioscope as part of their care.

He may have atrial fibrillation caused by mitral valve disease, carcinoma of the bronchus or thyrotoxicosis; heart block as a result of ischaemia; a chemical imbalance caused by an endocrine disorder or renal problems making him susceptible to dysrhythmias; ventricular dysrhythmias or bradycardia induced by drugs or paroxysmal supraventricular tachycardia caused by Wolff—Parkinson—White syndrome.

All these conditions deserve the best facilities for treatment that modern medicine can offer; however, the equipment is only as efficient as the operator.

4. Resuscitation

Death following collapse caused by cardiac arrest in hospital occurs less frequently as doctors and nurses learn to recognize the condition and to react quickly. Cardiac arrest is sudden cessation of circulation caused by absence of electrical activity (asystole, Fig. 4.1) or rapid bizarre electrical activity in the ventricles resulting in twitching movements with no effective cardiac output (ventricular fibrillation, Fig. 4.2).

As the nurse spends more time in the ward than the doctor she is more likely to notice sudden change in a patient's condition. If he has collapsed she has to decide quickly whether it is her duty to resuscitate. Some wards employ a code system to inform nurses but usually there is a well established method. General indications for resuscitation include patients who collapse post-operatively, after a myocardial infarction, undiagnosed patients, or normally healthy individuals admitted for a minor complaint.

If a decision is made to resuscitate the nurse should act quickly as the brain cells will only survive for three to four minutes once circulation has ceased. Observe him: he may be very pale or blue as he may have also stopped breathing and he may convulse or twitch. Confirm the diagnosis by feeling for a pulse. Find a major artery such as the carotid or femoral as the radial artery may be weak and difficult to feel if the patient has only a fainting attack.

Once the diagnosis is made (within seconds) call for help, using an emergency bell if one is at hand, but do not waste time. Start external cardiac massage and assisted mouth-to-mouth ventilation until help and equipment arrive.

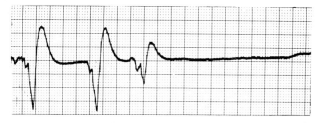

Fig. 4.1. After three bizarre ventricular beats there is asystole.

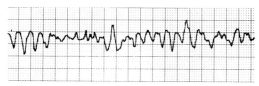

Fig. 4.2. Ventricular fibrillation.

On a Coronary Care Unit diagnosis is less of a problem because the patient is already attached to a cardiac monitor. There may be a warning rhythm change such as sudden bursts of self-terminating ventricular tachycardia, or the rhythm may suddenly become ventricular fibrillation (see Fig. 4.2).

The circulation ceases and the patient loses consciousness within five to 30 seconds. If a defibrillator is not immediately available the nurse and her team must start external cardiac massage, assisted ventilation and summon medical help.

In a well-organized unit there is often no need for cardiac massage. An alarm or observation quickly alerts the nurses. By the time the defibrillator is wheeled to the bedside and prepared for use, the patient should be lying flat on his back, hopefully unconscious and prepared for defibrillation, all within thirty seconds.

But care must be taken not to start resuscitative measures only on the evidence of the cardioscope. 'Asystole' may be produced when a monitoring electrode or wire becomes detached as a straight line is seen on the cardioscope. Ventricular fibrillation can be mimicked by a patient scratching an electrode, or vigorous movement of the patient cable (Fig. 4.3).

Conversely, do not assume a patient with a cardioscope show-

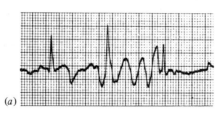

(a)

Fig. 4.3. (a) Regular sinus rhythm with superimposed artefact which makes it look similar to record (b) which consists mainly of multifocal ventricular tachycardia needing urgent treatment.

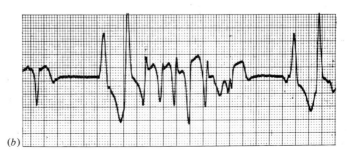

(b)

ing sinus rhythm has a good circulation. He may be effectively
dead (Fig. 4.4).

The rhythm strip in Fig. 4.4 was recorded from a man who
collapsed a few days after a myocardial infarction. Resuscitation
was unsuccessful and at post mortem he was found to have a
ruptured heart. Although the conducting system was working well
the ventricles were unable to circulate the blood. This is termed
electro-mechanical dissociation.

Diagnosis

Some points on diagnosis have already been made in earlier chapters. It cannot be over-stressed how important the time factor is
to the chances of the patient making a full recovery. Residual
brain damage or consequent renal failure may follow through pro-
longed hypoxia and hypotension if too little is done too late;
there is no gain, and a disservice has been done to the patient, his
family and health resources.

If the patient is found to be pulseless then cardiac arrest must
be assumed to have occurred. Do not waste time in attaching a
cardioscope to make the diagnosis. Cardiac massage alone may
stimulate the heart to beat if it is asystolic. Profound bradycardia
may cause circulatory collapse which could be reversed by cardiac
massage until other measures are available, such as stimulatory
drugs or the insertion of a pacemaker wire (Fig. 4.5).

Staff

Every ward has patients who may conceivably experience cardiac
arrest, however unlikely it may seem, and should be properly
staffed to deal with it. A junior nurse is just as able to begin

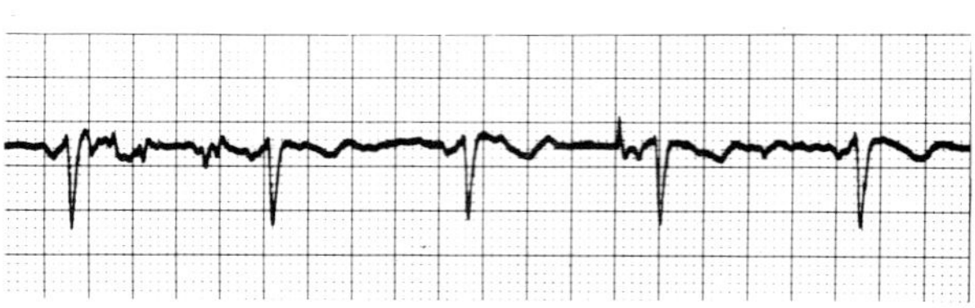

Fig. 4.4. Electromech-
anical dissociation.
This rhythm strip was
recorded from a patient
who was effectively
dead as there were no
mechanical events in
the heart — only
electric events. A
simultaneous pressure
trace would be flat.

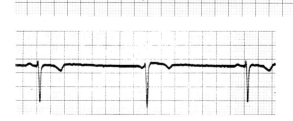

Fig. 4.5. Profound
bradycardia.

resuscitation as a qualified doctor if she is given the confidence through training. Nurses in specialized monitoring areas are trained, to a greater or lesser degree, to treat cardiac arrest. All are taught the initial measures to support the patient until the medical team arrives. More experienced nurses and those undergoing courses are taught to use the defibrillator, and to give some drugs. Others are also trained to intubate. Often a certificate of competence is issued signed by the senior nurse and medical consultant. The nurse accepts the responsibility to perform a challenging and rewarding procedure.

Equipment

Every ward or patient area should have an emergency box in an accessible position. A good idea employed on some wards is to keep a Brook airway or similar device in a polythene bag at the Sister's desk. The nurse becomes familiar with its presence and it enables her to start effective assisted ventilation, giving a better air entry with less danger of obstruction. All the nurses, not merely Sister or staff nurse, should be familiar with the contents of the box and involved in checking them regularly. The box will contain at least the basics:

several sizes of airway
a Brook oropharangeal airway
Ambubag and mask
mouth gag to prise the teeth apart
a laryngoscope with spare bulb and batteries
several sizes of intubation tube
Cobbs adaptor and catheter mount to fit Ambubag
introducer
KY jelly
Magill forceps (to remove obstructions and help guide the tube)
5 ml syringe for inflating the tube cuff
tape to tie the tube in place
stimulant drugs, including atropine, adrenaline, calcium chloride, calcium gluconate and isoprenaline
antiarrhythmic drugs, including lignocaine, propranolol
assorted syringes and needles

After checking and replenishing the box it should be sealed with tape which is easily broken when needed but it will also be obvious if the box has been opened at other times, perhaps with the removal of a vital piece of equipment. A lock would waste time.

More expensive equipment, such as cardioscopes and defibrillator, can be shared between groups of wards. It should be kept in a readily accessible unlocked area.

In a monitoring area, such as a Coronary Care Unit, the equipment is more refined. The patient is attached to a monitor which is protected against the voltage discharged from the defibrillator. The defibrillator is often mounted on a purpose-built trolley with drawers and cupboards for emergency equipment (Fig. 4.6).

The defibrillator should be placed centrally in the Unit with ready access to all patients at all times. Extra equipment, such as X-ray machines, must not be left in the area causing an obstruction.

Fig. 4.6. A purpose built trolley for the defibrillator and resuscitation equipment (St. Mary's Hospital, I.T.U., Paddington).

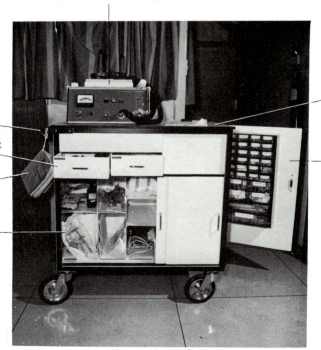

difibrillator mounted at an angle for ease of access to controls

paddles and cream stowed but ready for instant use

working su

pushing/pulling handle

Labelled drawers do not obstruct shelves below

cupboard, door for st needles, sy and drugs

daily checking book

labelled compartments for all accessories with sliding doors

fully mobile wheels with no brakes for instant manoeuverability

Using the defibrillator

The defibrillator is a device which administers a chosen amount of electrical energy, measured in joules (J) or watt seconds (J = W × s), through a pair of paddle-shaped electrodes. One paddle is placed on the chest above the heart and the other below the heart near the normal apex beat so that the current passes through the heart along its greatest axis reaching the largest area of heart muscle from base to apex.

Ventricular fibrillation is interrupted by a high energy shock of short duration so that all cells are depolarized causing all activity in the heart to cease. The sinus node pacemaker should recover most swiftly so the heart can restart at its proper rate and rhythm. If no activity is present in the heart the administration of an electric shock may stimulate it to restart.

When ventricular fibrillation occurs a nurse who can use the defibrillator, wheels it to the bedside, plugs in the electric cable and switches on the machine. She then takes the paddles, removes the rubber protective covers (if any) and squeezes a large blob of electrode jelly on to one paddle and rubs the paddle faces together to spread it quickly and evenly. The correct amount of energy is set (see later) and the dial is checked to ensure it registers.

Meanwhile the area is screened off and the patient prepared. Initially he may not be completely unconscious so he may hear what is said. He will be lying on a bed with a firm base. If a pillow happens to lie beneath his shoulders leave it as it helps to extend the neck, giving a clear airway. Remove all other pillows and undo the pyjama buttons or lift the nightdress to expose the chest. A sharp blow on the sternum with the fist may interrupt ventricular fibrillation or asystole and revert it to sinus rhythm. Both the patient and the defibrillator operator are now ready.

Ensure the patient is unconscious and look to see that no one is touching the bed or patient. Place the paddles on the chest above and below the heart along its greatest axis (see Fig. 4.7).

If the patient is very large it is safer to ask an assistant to hold the second paddle on the opposite side of the body rather than risk leaning over and touching him. Holding the paddles very firmly in place, press the button or buttons on the paddles to discharge the electricity. Look at the monitor. The trace should reappear on the cardioscope within three seconds. After a short period of asystole the patient's rhythm may return to normal, so he will quickly regain consciousness (Fig. 4.8).

Fig. 4.7. Placement of
paddles for emergency
defibrillation.

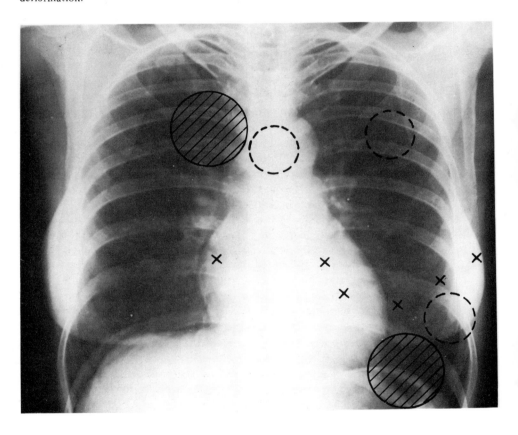

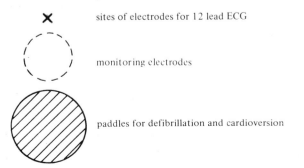

✕   sites of electrodes for 12 lead ECG

(   )   monitoring electrodes

◯   paddles for defibrillation and cardioversion

Check the pulse at the femoral artery to ensure that there is a good cardiac output. Assisted ventilation is not usually required but sometimes the patient needs encouragement and stimulation to breathe. Oxygen is usually given for a short while by face mask until any hypoxia has been corrected by the restored circulation. Medication, or other measures (such as pacing) may be taken to prevent further ventricular fibrillation. When heart rhythm is stabilized and blood pressure reasonable the patient may be sat up. Often the patient is unaware that anything more than a 'faint' has occurred. Sometimes, particularly if it happens several times, or if he was not fully unconscious, he is aware of a 'kick' in the chest and soreness, but most patients readily accept a brief, factual explanation. Other patients in the unit usually find a successful defibrillation encouraging.

Recurrent ventricular fibrillation

After the first electric shock the cardioscope may still show ventricular fibrillation, so a second shock is required. A few seconds are needed to re-apply jelly to the paddles and to recharge the defibrillator, perhaps to a higher level. Meanwhile the second nurse should perform external cardiac massage and, if time or if more help is available, assisted ventilation with added oxygen. If both these procedures are very effective the patient may become more conscious, so it is kinder to allow him a few seconds to lapse into unconsciousness prior to further defibrillation. If the second attempt is ineffective it is essential to continue with cardiac massage and assisted ventilation until medical help arrives. Further electric shocks will be ineffective and produce more cardiac damage, so wait until metabolic acidosis has been corrected by an infusion of sodium bicarbonate, when defibrillation may become effective.

Fig. 4.8. Ventricular fibrillation reverts to pacing rhythm after defibrillation.

Sometimes defibrillation results in asystole in which case continue with cardiac massage and assisted ventilation, having summoned medical aid.

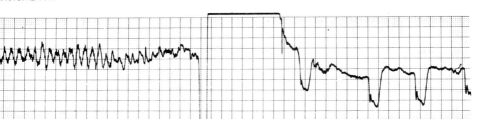

More detail is needed on some points and there are various other aspects to consider which will be dealt with under separate headings.

The trolley

A trolley constructed for individual units is probably most satisfactory (see Fig. 4.6). It takes time to evolve the ideal design as it depends on such factors as space available in the unit and the preferences of various doctors, e.g. choice of drugs.

Ensure the trolley, fully equipped, is light enough to move easily. If it is large a handle at either end is useful. Wheels should be fully mobile so that it can be readily moved in any direction. No brakes should be fitted.

The defibrillator should be placed on the trolley so that all the controls can be seen unobstructed. Nothing should be stored over ventilator grills. The paddles should be mounted safely already plugged in for instant use. Drawers and cupboards should not obstruct one another. Sliding doors are useful when space is at a premium. Store different items in separate compartments as far as possible, e.g. equipment for defibrillation in one area, intubation equipment in another and stimulant drugs with syringes and needles elsewhere. A tray for intubation equipment is useful as it can be moved quickly to the head of the bed. If there is room, extra equipment can be kept in various compartments, including intravenous equipment, intracardiac needles, spare monitoring electrodes, a thorocotomy pack and tracheostomy pack.

Electric cables, particularly the mains, must be free to be plugged in immediately. A spring clip is useful for holding the coiled cable, avoiding time spent in unwinding it. If an ambubag is attached to the trolley it is best placed where it cannot be squashed against a wall and burst in the rush. A rubbish bag and box for sharps is helpful in keeping the area organized. A flat surface incorporated into the trolley, such as a sliding shelf, is useful as a drug checking area or for writing when working space is limited.

Daily checking

This is an essential routine and any faults should be dealt with as an emergency. Check that all wired connections are secure, and that there are no splits in the cable covering. If the machine has to be taken for repair or servicing, insist that the firm or hospital will offer a similar model on loan. Check lists should be kept with the trolley for easy reference. Ensure all equipment is clean and ready for use. Safety for patient, operator and others at the scene relies on proper checking procedures, regular maintenance and correct use of the machine. The operator should be thoroughly trained by a competent person and be able to accept and discharge the responsibility.

The defibrillator
There are many designs available so each patient area can choose an appropriate machine. Some are mains-operated, some battery, and others both.

In a high-dependence area it is useful to have a standby battery-operated machine as the mains defibrillator may already be in use, develop a fault or there may be a power cut. A battery model should be available for transferring a patient from the admission area or to the operating theatre. It is strongly recommended that a charging unit is permanently connected when not in use. This should have an on/off light indicator and it should be attached firmly enough so that it cannot easily be dislodged, interrupting charging. After using or checking a battery defibrillator, ensure the off switch is used even though the paddles have been discharged, or they will continue to draw power and flatten the battery.

One type of battery defibrillator can dishcarge forty times at 400 J, and takes ten seconds to recharge to a maximum level of 400 J. There is an automatic safety circuit to prevent a higher energy being discharged. It has a priming button which causes a light to glow for ten seconds during which time the electricity can be discharged. If unused the charge automatically shorts out so, if needed, it must be reprimed. A battery low warning light shines when five charges at 400 J each are left. It can be used for synchronized defibrillation. At 19.5 kg (43 lb), it is rather heavy for a nurse to carry easily.

Smaller defibrillators are available which are more manageable. Another defibrillator incorporates a pair of paddles attached by sprung cables to an electrical unit containing a battery. These are particularly useful for the situation when the equipment must be taken away from a mains source, e.g. into the hospital grounds or corridors.

In a group of wards or a nursing home where a cardiac arrest is uncommon a shared mobile defibrillator is a useful asset; although initially expensive, it may save a few lives.

A further design of defibrillator is produced which is mains or battery operated and is supposedly portable but very heavy. A carrying handle converts to a stand while it is in use. Dry electrodes can be placed on the chest and the rhythm is picked up by the paddles and appears on a screen. The write-out is often of poor quality, however. Picture size on the cardioscope can be adjusted by moving a switch on to position 1, 2 or 3, and there is a freeze button. The same electrodes are used for defibrillation up to 400 J. Write-out facilities are available and a two-way radio telephone can be attached so the doctor can contact the emergency admission area. When not in use it should be kept on constant charge. The cable supplied is designed to fit well into the socket on the defibrillator and cannot easily fall out. When fully charged the battery lasts for eight hours.

The paediatric model of the last defibrillator described is similar but the amount of energy available is 320 J. The paddles have smaller electrode areas but the handles are the same as for adults with a good-sized shield so they are easily manageable.

Permanent cardiac damage can be caused if too much energy is delivered, so particular care must be taken with babies and children. Recommended dosage for them is:

2.2 J/kg (body weight) for ventricular fibrillation.
1.5 J/kg (body weight) for ventricular tachycardia and supra-
    ventricular tachycardia.

Several large cities operate a Coronary Ambulance which is summoned when someone collapses in the street or place of work. These are generally well equipped and use battery-operated devices.

In some hospitals large, older models of defibrillator are used which are heavy and difficult to manoeuvre and need a lift to move them from floor to floor. Although still useful they are perhaps best kept in areas where they do not need to be moved far. Many have developed wiring faults by now, so get electrical experts to check over old machines that you see in use.

Electrical energy
The electrical energy discharged is converted from the mains alternating current to direct current so that a precise amount of

energy is delivered to the patient. 400 J is the maximum energy used. Some machines incorporate a dial so that a variable amount of energy can be used while others have a graduated dial which is set to a particular number. When using the defibrillator, if the dial shows more energy than is required, it is quicker to discharge it and start again than to wait for a little to leak away. Some models employ a leak button to allow the loss of a controlled amount of charge. When checking the machine, charge it to a small number of joules, e.g. 10 J, and check that this amount registers. If the indicating needle moves much beyond it or if the current leaks out quickly before it is discharged, it needs attention.

When treating ventricular fibrillation in adults the usual amount of current used initially is 200–300 J, increasing to 400 J maximum if that is ineffective. When a patient suffers from persistent bouts of ventricular fibrillation the smallest successful amount of energy such as 100–150 J should be used. Other factors that govern the amount used are the size of the patient and whether the patient is digitalized.

Synchronized shock (cardioversion)

Normally, for emergency purposes the defibrillator is set to discharge electricity immediately the buttons on the paddles are pressed. However, many machines can also be set up in the synchronized mode (often called 'cardiovert') to discharge only on the downstroke of the R wave (Fig. 4.9) and so avoid the T wave, i.e. during ventricular repolarization. This is the 'vulnerable' period of the cardiac cycle when the electricity in the cells of the myocardium and conducting system is stabilizing ready for the next contraction. If another electrical source fires during this phase ventricular fibrillation may ensue (see Fig. 1.2).

The synchronized mode (cardioversion) is used when a patient has a rhythm disturbance which is disadvantageous but not necessarily life-threatening. If not adequately treated soon enough, such

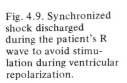
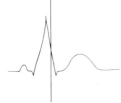

Fig. 4.9. Synchronized shock discharged during the patient's R wave to avoid stimulation during ventricular repolarization.

dysrhythmias, especially following myocardial infarction, may
endanger life. Drugs are available but it is often quicker, has less
side effects and is more permanent, if a defibrillator is used. Such
dysrhythmias include supraventricular tachycardia (Fig. 4.10),
atrial fibrillation and atrial flutter which may be either slowed by
drugs to a more normal ventricular rate or, preferably, converted
to normal sinus rhythm by cardioversion (Fig. 4.11). Whatever
the ventricular rate, these dysrhythmias lead to loss of normal
atrial transport function, filling the ventricles at end-diastole. If
it persists cardiac output falls and the patient may become hypotensive and hypoxic, especially if there is a tachycardia or if the
myocardium is damaged. Rarely the patient becomes unconscious.
Usually synchronized cardioversion is an elective procedure so

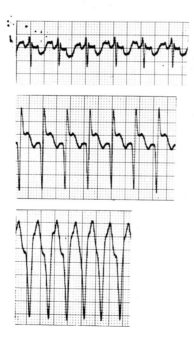

Fig. 4.10. Recordings
of three types of supra-
ventricular tachycardia
that may be treated by
cardioversion.

Fig. 4.11. Supra-
ventricular tachycardia
is reverted to sinus
rhythm with right
bundle branch block
(lead MCL1) by
cardioversion.

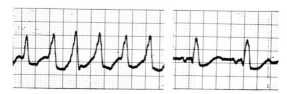

the patient signs a consent form, the doctor having explained the procedure. If the patient is digitalized it is usual to withdraw digoxin for at least 24 hours prior to cardioversion (see note on digoxin). Dentures and spectacles are removed and he lies flat on his back on a hard-based bed, with chest bared. If hirsute, it is advisable to shave the patch where the paddles will be placed. An anaesthetist must be present to give a brief anaesthetic and he checks that equipment is at hand if intubation is necessary.

The patient is attached to a cardiac monitor to which the defibrillator is connected via a long lead. Usually the same make of equipment is used but in some cases a special adaptor module is needed. Set the defibrillator to the synchronized mode so that each R wave is recognized by the machine. On some machines the tracing can be increased in size until a light flashes on each R wave. The anaesthetist gives the patient a short acting sedative, e.g. i.v. althesin or i.v. valium. When the patient is unconscious the pre-jelled paddles are pressed firmly on the chest. The button(s) is pressed and held until the electricity is dishcarged automatically by the R wave, avoiding a T wave and the vulnerable period.

As the electricity is not immediately discharged it is important to continue to press the paddles firmly on the chest, as premature release of pressure will result in the electricity arcing, i.e. it will flash across the chest from one paddle to another. This wastes some of the voltage and may burn the chest. As only small amounts of electricity are used for cardioversion (10–100 J) the lost current may mean a second shock is required with continuing sedation.

Often the dysrhythmia slows or reverts to normal after one shock but sometimes a series of shocks is needed, increasing the energy each time. After a previously decided amount is given the procedure may be stopped if it is unsuccessful and the patient allowed to regain consciousness. He is turned on to his side and a nurse stays with him until he is conscious. An oral airway may be needed initially.

Ventricular tachycardia
If a patient who has poor myocardial function or is hypotensive develops rapid ventricular tachycardia (Fig. 4.12), he may become unconscious and should be treated as for cardiac arrest. The defibrillator is used in the non-synchronized mode for speed as some machines take a minute or so to set up for synchronized

shock. Because of this he may possibly develop ventricular fibrillation when a second shock would be needed.

Asystole
A doctor finding a patient asystolic sometimes uses a large shock from a defibrillator to attempt to stimulate the heart. It is reasonable to do this if the patient is pulseless prior to attaching a cardioscope as the few seconds saved could be vital and ventricular fibrillation is the common cause of arrest. It is policy on some units to shock an asystolic heart in the hope of stimulating it.

Digoxin
Digoxin lowers the threshold of ventricular ectopics so that ventricular fibrillation is more likely to occur, especially if there is a stimulus, such as the shock delivered from a defibrillator, even when synchronized, so when administering shocks to a digitalized patient it should be done with great caution.
Ensure he is not digoxin-toxic, check the potassium level to ensure he is not hypokalaemic, premedicate with an antidysrhythmic drug, e.g. lignocaine, and use very low energy shocks. It is the policy of some units that no patient should receive digoxin after a myocardial infarction.

If a patient suffers from digoxin toxicity, which may produce bursts of ventricular tachycardia or ventricular fibrillation, it is advisable to admit him to a monitoring unit so that appropriate therapy can be given to prevent ventricular fibrillation.

Paddles
Usually adult-sized paddles for external defibrillation are attached for instant use. One paddle only may have a discharge button, but often there is one on each for additional safety. If there are two buttons they are pressed simultaneously to discharge the current. A pair of paddles is available which have a

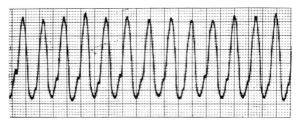

Fig. 4.12. Ventricular tachycardia.

built-in cushion under the electrode plate. The current is only discharged when the operator presses the paddles sufficiently hard against the chest. The metal electrode surface area is about 10 cm in diameter mounted in plastic insulated handles with a guard between the handle and electrode plate. The guard is designed to protect the operator if the electrodes are damp but will conduct electricity if electrode jelly is smeared on the handle between the plate and the operator's hands. The operator should ensure that she has clean dry hands and should use an economical amount of jelly which will not drip off the plates but is sufficient to cover them completely so the patient is not burnt.

Paediatric paddles are available which have a smaller electrode area (40 mm) and plug into the usual defibrillator. If the defibrillator is supplied with paediatric paddles these should also be stored in the trolley.

Intracardiac paddles for use in direct contact with the heart look very different. They have a smaller surface area which is curved like spoons to fit snugly against the heart with direct contact. They are covered in soft metallic material. They are kept in cardio-thoracic theatres, and emergency areas such as the admission area or Coronary Care Unit also often keep intracardiac paddles in a sealed sterile container, in case open defibrillation is needed, but this is rarely justified now that external defibrillation is so successful.

The paddles normally used with the machine are checked as part of the daily schedule. Often a specially insulated plate is fitted to the trolley or defibrillator on which the paddles can be mounted. They can be left *in situ* while the discharge button is pressed for testing. Never hold the paddle faces together when testing unless the manufacturer particularly recommends this.

External paddles are washed in warm soapy water, rinsed and dried thoroughly. They should not be immersed in water. Internal paddles are usually sterilized in the hospital's Central Sterile Supplies Department, by autoclaving. The cables are sterilized separately in an ethylene oxide chamber.

Jelly
The electrode jelly used is the same type used for taking an electro-cardiogram. It acts as a conducting medium and protects the skin from an electrical burn. Some are more fluid than others but a creamy consistency is best for use with a defibrillator as it is more controllable and less likely to run and splash. Replace the tube

before it becomes half empty to avoid delays in squeezing the jelly out. Ensure the cap is firmly replaced to prevent the jelly drying out. Paper towels or swabs are useful to wipe excess jelly from the chest between defibrillations, and will prevent current being lost by conduction across it. If repeated shocks are needed ensure the electrode plates are well-covered each time. Do not allow jelly to dry on the paddles or on the chest as it will burn the patient. Wipe excess jelly off the chest before starting cardiac massage to avoid skidding off the sternum with the possibility of breaking ribs.

Pads of conducting gel are available for use with a defibrillator. A set of two is packaged in a sealed envelope to prevent drying out. The pads feel sticky to touch and some need separating by pulling apart at a perforated line. A set of pads can be used for repeated defibrillations on a patient.

Disposable electrodes for defibrillation can also be used. These are large circular discs with contact jelly on the side to be placed on the patient. The upper surface has a metallic surface on which the paddles are placed.

Both the above products are probably quicker to use than applying electrode jelly but they would seem to encourage multiple shocks over the same two areas of the chest, which should be discouraged in the interest of skin care. Also there is the danger of dry electrodes being applied which would burn and time would be wasted in applying new pads. However, they are effective and, used with awareness, they are time-saving and less messy.

Gloves
Rubber gloves were once worn routinely by the operator for insulation but it is no longer thought to be necessary. Clean, dry hands are better. Vital seconds are lost in putting them on. Paddle handles are well insulated so, if they are held correctly using the hand shield, accidents are prevented. Ensure the hands are dry and free from jelly. An accident occurred while, unknown to the wearer, a glove was torn by an ampoule which was lodged in the finger. It smashed, causing the injection fluid to conduct current from the electrode to the operator who sustained a severe shock.

Skin care
One electric shock should cause no skin damage. If a geographical

burn appears on the skin this is caused by too little pressure on the paddles. If several shocks are needed, the skin should be wiped gently after each, if there is time. Dry jelly on the skin will conduct the electricity, thus spreading the burn. Place the paddles in a slightly different place each time, and keep the paddle faces well covered with jelly. Necrosis of the skin may occur if a large number of shocks over a short period is needed, but this can be minimized by proper care. Some proprietary burns creams are available which soothe the area.

Conscious or unconscious

If a doctor is present when ventricular fibrillation occurs he may not wait for the patient to be totally unconscious as the sooner the attempt to revert the rhythm the more successful it will be. Also hypoxia quickly occurs so brain cells will begin to die. A nurse may prefer to wait a few more seconds. When the shock is administered the muscle spasm may make the patient cry out. Often he will remember nothing but if he recalls the pain and discomfort reassurance is needed. Unless he is deeply unconscious the current will cause a reflex jerking movement which is worrying to the operator if not expected. The nurse who has the opportunity of using the defibrillator for the first time under the controlled conditions of cardioversion is fortunate. Others, who have accepted the responsibility, must rely on good teaching and observation. A teaching aid of a torso model is available which can be defibrillated when certain dysrhythmias appear on a screen. Unless it is used constantly and maintained properly, the cost is probably not justified — it is better to watch an experienced operator at work.

Place of arrest

Where a patient happens to arrest is not always convenient. He may be walking about in the ward, sitting in a chair or lying in bed. He is most accessible if lying on a bed that has a hard base and a removable head-rest. If he is in a chair, pull him down onto the floor, being careful of his head, as cardiac massage needs to be performed on a firm base. If the defibrillator is instantly available, defibrillate him initially while in the chair. Thereafter he can be lain on the floor for further resuscitation or if repeated shocks are needed.

As it is recognized that more lives can be saved and resuscitation becomes more effective, with better prospects of full recovery, more Coronary Care Units are used as monitoring areas for other patients at risk from cardiac arrest. Cardiac arrest can be prevented by careful monitoring and the administration of drugs to prevent myocardial irritability leading to ventricular fibrillation, or if bradycardia and heart blocks resulting in asystole are treated with a pacemaker. Electrolyte balance is carefully monitored. Patients with a metabolic disorder causing electrolyte imbalance, e.g. amyloid, may be nursed here. Procedures which may lead to ventricular irritability are performed under careful monitoring, e.g. aspiration of pericardial effusion.

The experienced personnel and expensive equipment may be used more effectively if the monitoring unit is made generally available for all patients at risk from cardiac dysrhythmias, but this may be a controversial viewpoint.

5. Pacemakers

The use of pacemakers in cardiology has increased enormously in recent years as new techniques are developed, more applications found for them and as doctors become more aware of their advantages.

A pacemaker is an electronic device (known also as a pulse generator) which stimulates the myocardium to contract using electrodes in contact with the heart (Fig. 5.1). The complete system consists of a generator in which the power supply is situated, and the electronic circuit and lead which takes the impulse to the myocardium. The current delivered depends upon the output of the pacemaker and the resistance (see Chapter 8) of the electrode and its contact with the myocardium. Each stimulus lasts from 0.05 to 2.0 ms.

A pacemaker can be a *demand unit*, inhibited by natural R waves and only stimulating the heart if no intrinsic beat occurs, or a *fixed rate unit* which fires constantly. Both facilities are sometimes available on one box for temporary pacing when special care must be taken not to change the mode accidentally.

Demand pacing

The pacing wire inserted into the ventricle delivers an electrical

Fig. 5.1. External pacing box, attachments and pacing wire.

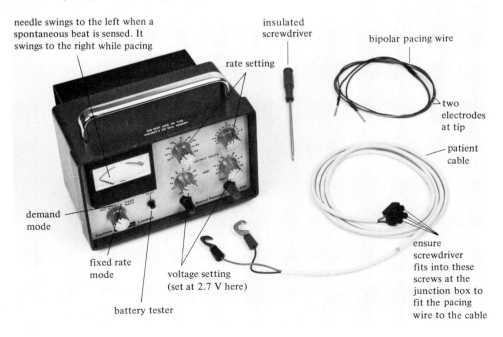

needle swings to the left when a spontaneous beat is sensed. It swings to the right while pacing

insulated screwdriver

bipolar pacing wire

rate setting

two electrodes at tip

patient cable

demand mode

fixed rate mode

voltage setting (set at 2.7 V here)

battery tester

ensure screwdriver fits into these screws at the junction box to fit the pacing wire to the cable stimulus to the heart and also senses when electrical activity has occurred. When a box is set 'on demand' it will only stimulate the heart if no activity is sensed within a pre-set time limit, which can be altered (Fig. 5.2). For example, if the box is set to fire on demand at 70 beats/min but the patient's heart rate is 80 beats/min the pacemaker will be inhibited. However, if his rate falls to 65 beats/min the pacemaker will produce stimulation to make up the difference. The facility to change the demand rate by one or two beats is useful when a patient has a spontaneous rate which is similar to that set on the pacemaker. If his blood pressure is rather low it may be improved by allowing the patient the benefit of atrial transport function with his own spontaneous but slightly slower heart rate, e.g. 65 beats/min.

Atrial transport function is sometimes termed atrial 'boost' or atrial 'kick'. The atria usually contract shortly before the ventricles and push about 30% of the total cardiac output (the stroke volume) into the ventricles. The ventricles, having received this amount of blood, contract to give a greater cardiac output and therefore act as a more efficient pump. If the atria fail to contract (e.g. during junctional rhythm) or contract in a rapid bizarre fashion (e.g. atrial fibrillation), or at a regular rate but not before each ventricular beat (e.g. during pacing, ventricular tachycardia or idioventricular rhythm), the cardiac output may fall and blood pressure may drop. The pacemaker can be set on demand at 60 beats/min and increased if it is found that he reverts to pacing for long periods. Then there is no possibility of a pacing beat and an intrinsic heart beat competing to cause a pacing impulse discharging on the T wave of the preceding beat with the risk of ventricular fibrillation (see Chapter 4). This complication is particularly likely in the sensitive ventricle after acute myocardial infarction and demand pacing is preferred in this situation.

Demand pacemakers are used in patients whose intrinsic rhythm is likely to recur or whose conduction problems are intermittent. Occasionally a paced beat occurs a few milliseconds after the initiation of a spontaneous beat so conduction is travelling simultaneously from two sources, therefore the myocardium

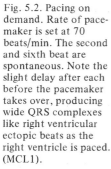

Fig. 5.2. Pacing on demand. Rate of pacemaker is set at 70 beats/min. The second and sixth beat are spontaneous. Note the slight delay after each before the pacemaker takes over, producing wide QRS complexes like right ventricular ectopic beats as the right ventricle is paced. (MCL1).

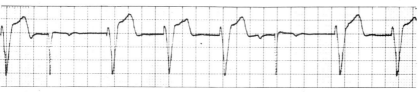

is stimulated more quickly. The resultant beat may be preceded by a P wave, there is a pacing artefact and the configuration is intermediate between both the normal beat and the paced beat. This is called a fusion beat and should be recognized so that it is not mistaken for an ectopic beat (Fig. 5.3).

Fixed-rate pacing

This system is used in patients whose intrinsic pacemaker has failed completely, perhaps through ischaemic damage or as a con-genital problem. It may also be used in elderly patients with degenerative complete heart block which has been established for a while.

A fixed-rate unit will stimulate the heart continuously at the rate set on the box. Spontaneous cardiac activity is usually sup-pressed but if it occurs, such as ectopic beats, it will be ignored.

If a patient has spontaneous rhythm and a fixed pacemaker triggers on the T wave, during the vulnerable period, there is danger of ventricular fibrillation.

External or internal units are used depending on the needs of the patient. The atria or ventricles may be paced individually or synchronously depending on the pacing equipment used.

External pacemakers

These are used temporarily for a number of hours, days or a few weeks. Many Coronary Care Units have facilities for inserting pacing electrodes as an emergency procedure if the patient is likely to become asystolic as a result of damage to the conducting system following a myocardial infarction. Most Units have strict criteria, decided by the consultant, so that junior doctors have no doubt when a pacing wire should be employed.

Controversy exists about prophylactic pacing for bundle branch blocks after myocardial infarction to prevent asystole, as it is not without dangers and significant decrease in mortality

Fig. 5.3. This ECG rhythm strip illustrates three types of QRS complex. On the left there are four com-plexes induced by the pacemaker. On the right are three natural complexes. The com-plex in the middle is an intermediate form, and is due partly to natural and partly to pacemaker conduction. It is known as a fusion beat.

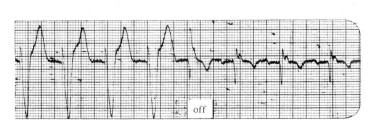

has not been proved. There is general agreement that it is advantageous to pace slow rhythms unresponsive to atropine although some doctors try isoprenaline first despite its hazards. The decision often depends on experience and the equipment available. If the patient has to be taken to another area for the operation the doctor will be reluctant to risk moving him in a critical condition when a pacemaker may save his life.

Once any of the following conditions develop there is danger of rapid deterioration to an asystolic cardiac arrest. If the rate is slow the already injured heart sustains more damage through hypoxia with increasing possibility of ventricular tachycardia and fibrillation.

Post myocardial infarct: usually inferior or posterior wall
(1) Severe sinus bradycardia which is unresponsive to atropine or to avoid giving repeated doses which may lead to toxicity.
(2) Second degree heart block with low ventricular rate (i.e. below 70 beats/min) with or without hypotension (Fig. 5.4). but unresponsive to atropine. Examples: (*a*) Mobitz type I atrio-ventricular block (Wenckebach); (*b*) 2:1 heart block.
(3) Complete heart block with a narrow ventricular complex. The rate may be good, 70–80 beats/min, but the condition is unstable and the rate may slow disastrously (Fig. 5.5).

Post myocardial infarct: anterior wall
(1) Complete heart block with wide complexes; the rate is often below 60 beats/min (Fig. 5.6).
(2) Left bundle branch block with first degree block (see Chapter 1).
(3) Right bundle branch block with left posterior hemiblock (see Chapter 1).
(4) Right bundle branch block with left anterior hemiblock and first degree heart block.

Fig. 5.4. Wenckebach rhythm, a second degree heart block, becomes 2:1 heart block after three P waves, resulting in a slow ventricular rate.

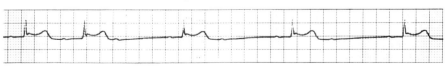

Fig. 5.5. Complete heart block; the complex is narrow and the heart rate is nearly normal.

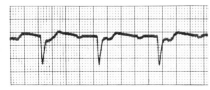

A temporary pacemaker is often helpful during anaesthesia and may be inserted pre-operatively for:

(a) Patients known to develop severe bradycardia during anaesthesia; (b) patients with bundle branch block (even if long standing). It is often used prophylactically after open heart surgery.

Outpacing a tachydysrhythmia is a useful recent development. An electrode wire is sited in the right atrium or right ventricle or both to stimulate either or both chambers to beat at a greater rate than the dysrhythmia, which may be supraventricular or ventricular in origin.

Bradycardias, induced by drug overdosage can be treated with a temporary pacemaker.

A patient needing a permanent pacemaker may have a temporary unit initially if theatre space is not immediately available and he is experiencing Adam Stoke's attacks.

Diagnostic uses of temporary pacing

The tip of the wire may be sited to stimulate the right atrium. Although it is difficult to achieve stable atrial pacing, it is possible to lodge the tip in the coronary sinus or in the atrial appendage. It is usually only needed temporarily while studies are undertaken:

(1) to study conduction through the atrio-ventricular node and bundle of His (the junction of the heart). The atria can be paced very rapidly, then the stimulation is suddenly stopped to study the spontaneous recovery and function of the sino-atrial node.

(2) to increase the heart rate to produce cardiac stress in patients with coronary artery disease or ischaemia. Pain threshold, and electrocardiographic, haemodynamic and biochemical changes can be studied.

(3) to deliver premature beats in order to provoke tachydysrhythmias and to stop them. The timing of paced beats needed to terminate the tachycardia can be studied so that a pacing

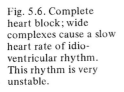

Fig. 5.6. Complete heart block; wide complexes cause a slow heart rate of idio-ventricular rhythm. This rhythm is very unstable.

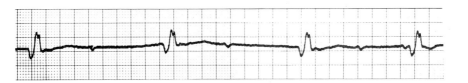

unit delivering timed stimuli can be designed for a patient
with a specific rhythm disturbance.

(4) to study the site of origin of an irritable focus prior to possible surgery to destroy it.

Insertion of a temporary pacing wire
With a reasonably co-operative patient and good equipment the
procedure is simple in competent hands.

Basically an insulated wire with two electrodes at the tip
(bipolar) is inserted into a major vein to enter the heart through
the right atrium, passing through the tricuspid valve, to sit in the
apex of the right ventricle.

The sites of entry are:

(*a*) the subclavian vein, right and left;

(*b*) the internal jugular vein, right and left;

(*c*) the cephalic vein at the right or left antecubital fossa;

(*d*) via the right or left femoral vein (rarely);

(*e*) intracardiac (as an emergency). This is rarely used.

(*f*) post-cardiac surgery; the wire is routinely placed against the
ventricle during the operation, protruding through or near the
stitch line.

Equipment. The patient lies on a radio-translucent bed. An image
intensifier X-ray machine scans the chest to demonstrate the progress of the wire throughout the procedure, displaying the picture
on a television screen. It is useful to keep an emergency sterile
pacing pack laid on a trolley. The following equipment is needed
on the trolley.

(i) Sterile towels:

one large to place under the patient;

one small to wrap round the patient's head to cover the hair;

one small placed on the handle of the image intensifier to
enable the doctor to move it, if necessary;

two or three medium towels to place around the operation
site;

waterproof sheet to lie under the patient.

(ii) Solutions:

sodium chloride, 0.9% for injection, or dextrose saline;

skin cleansing solution.

(iii) Local anaesthetic: lignocaine 1%, marcaine 0.5% or 0.25%,
or citanest 1%.

(iv) Instruments:

two gallipots;

sponge-holding forceps;
2 ml syringe with large and small needle;
scalpel handle and blade or stylet;
introduction cannula (wide bore needle with plastic guide);
suture-holding forceps;
scissors;
toothed forceps;
skin suture and needle;
gauze swabs;
strapping.

The patient. A consent form is usual in all but dire emergencies. Explanation of the procedure will help the patient to co-operate.

Remove his upper clothing to expose the neck area and chest. Check that monitoring electrodes will not impede the view of the heart or obstruct the site of electrode insertion. Resite any that may. Shave the operation site if necessary for ease of access and to minimize the risk of infection. Many doctors like to insert a temporary intravenous cannula, if no infusion is in progress, to give immediate therapy if necessary. Ensure that oxygen tubing does not impede the operation site or view of the chest. Use tape to keep it out of the way if it is essential for the patient to have oxygen. Remove spectacles, but there is no need to remove dentures unless he is at particular risk. Some patients experience difficulty in talking without dentures. If the patient has a troublesome cough a draught of cough suppressant would be helpful and a glass of water with a flexible straw kept at the bedside. Sedation is rarely necessary and could prolong the procedure if the patient is unable to co-operate in moving or coughing. If sedation is essential before operating is possible, the risk of airway obstruction must be considered and measures taken to prevent it.

Arrangement of equipment. The patient lies on a radio-translucent bed. Remove all extras from the bed such as foot cradle or surplus intravenous stands and clear any obstructions from under the bed so that the image intensifier can be manoeuvred to swing freely across the chest. Place the television screen where the doctor can easily watch the progress of the wire.

A trolley laid with sterile pacing equipment is placed next to the doctor who stands at the head of the bed on the patient's right side. If he uses a femoral approach or enters a vein on the patient's left the equipment is reversed. An assistant stands at the opposite side of the trolley. Both wear sterile gloves, caps, masks

and gowns. The cardioscope is placed so that the doctor can see
it and a nurse or technician is assigned to watch the monitor continuously throughout the procedure and to report dysrhythmias.
Place the defibrillator so that it does not obstruct other equipment but is accessible for instant use. Set it up for direct use but
with no jelly on the paddles as it will dry out.

The pacemaker box is checked to ensure the battery is effective and in date, and the two leads are firmly attached. If there is
a junction box the screws are loosened ready to receive the
pacing wire. Using the screwdriver before the procedure begins
ensures it fits. The screwdriver is kept near the box.

Check that the pacing wire is functioning by attaching it to a
circuit testing box with an ammeter which will register the
amount of current which flows. Re-sterilize the tips which
touched the circuit testing box by immersing them in the cleansing fluid. A gauze pad placed over the tips in the solution will
help prevent them from falling out of the gallipot. Check that the
wire will easily pass through the plastic guide. Ensure the wire is
not too mobile.

Set the rate on the pacemaker so that it is greater than the
patient's with the voltage on 3 V so it is ready to switch on
instantly.

Check that everyone in the vicinity is wearing a lead apron,
then switch on the X-ray equipment to ensure it works, giving a
clear image that occupies the entire screen. Always switch on at
the mains before switching on the individual parts of the
machine.

The procedure. The skin is cleaned with a non-electrostatic fluid,
a waterproof sheet with a sterile towel over it is placed under the
patient and sterile towels are placed around the operation site.
The vein is located and the skin around it is injected with local
anaesthetic, first with a small bore needle, then a wider needle
for deeper anaesthesia. A tiny incision is made near the vein with
a scalpel blade or stylet and a 2 ml syringe containing sodium
chloride 0.9% or dextrose saline is inserted into the vein with a
plastic guide covering the needle. The syringe may need to be disconnected from the needle several times to flush out the blood
and refilled with intravenous fluid until the exact position is
found. Once the vein is entered the syringe and needle are withdrawn, leaving the plastic guide through which the pacing electrode passes.

The arm of the X-ray apparatus is swung across the patient's chest and moved higher or lower as necessary. Lighting around the patient is dimmed or switched off and adjustments made to brightness or focus as on a normal television set. If the patient is obese a more penetrating image will be needed. Once the image is good the doctor advances the electrode wire, watching the screen and feeling the progress of the wire. Meanwhile an experienced person looks at the cardioscope. A system should be evolved to inform the doctor of any dangerous cardiac activity, such as calling 'one' for each ectopic initially, 'VT' for ventricular tachycardia (three or more ventricular ectopics together) or 'VF' for ventricular fibrillation. Asystole is another complication if the patient has a total left bundle branch block and the right bundle fails either coincidentally or as a result of damage by the wire. A few atrial ectopics are often noted as the wire moves across the right atrium.

If there are numerous ventricular ectopics or bursts of ventricular tachycardia it is advisable for the doctor to stop to allow the irritation to settle. Lignocaine 2%, or another intravenous anti-dysrhythmic agent, may be helpful if the activity is excessive and continuous infusion may be needed. If an infusion of isoprenaline is in progress before pacing this is usually discontinued prior to the procedure as it is a myocardial irritant.

It is normal to note a few right ventricular ectopics as the wire enters the ventricle. Care is taken to place the tip as near the apex of the right ventricle as possible to minimize the risk of dislodging the wire and to give the lowest threshold for pacing. It lodges in amongst the trabeculae carneae. Once it seems to be well sited the terminals are attached to the junction box or directly on to the pacemaker. The voltage is checked, the rate set so that it is greater than the patient's rate, and the box switched on to demand pacing. On the cardioscope the patient's rhythm should be replaced by regular pacing artefacts followed by a paced beat each time. This is termed 'capture'. Right ventricular ectopics may be present but these usually settle quickly. If persistent after re-positioning the wire a lignocaine infusion may be needed temporarily.

The threshold is checked before suturing. This establishes the least amount of electricity required to pace the heart. Ensure that the rhythm is continuous pacing. Increase the rate if the patient's own rhythm competes. Pace at 2 V or 3 V then, using the fine scale, slowly decrease the voltage until there is continuous pacing at 1 V. Turn the fine scale to register 1 V again and reduce the other to zero so that pacing at 1 V continues. Decrease the fine scale by 0.1 V at a time until the point is reached when the patient's intrinsic rhythm occurs, demonstrating when capture is lost. This is the threshold, usually about 0.1–0.9 V. If asystole occurs the pacemaker must be set at a greater voltage immediately to recommence pacing. The closer the contact with endocardium the lower the threshold will be and less electricity will be needed. If too great a voltage is delivered there is danger of causing ventricular fibrillation. At least twice the threshold is set on the box but 2 V or 3 V is usual to allow for slight movement of the electrode catheter and for 'inflammation' around the tip of the catheter, which may impede conduction a little.

Once a good pacing position is established the wire is stitched to the skin, using sutures firmly tied to the wire so that it cannot be dislodged. The patient is asked to deep breathe and cough at intervals during the suturing to ensure it remains *in situ*. Once stitched the threshold is re-checked. The skin is cleaned and dried and a small pad of sterile gauze is placed over the stitches. Coil the wire freely in wide loops over the shoulder, if the subclavian or internal jugular veins are used, so there is no risk of fracture, and strap it firmly with the junction box protruding towards the arm, for access and patient comfort.

Often a larger type of pacemaker box is used initially as there is a needle which swings across when a pacing beat is delivered. Some models have a dial with a needle in the centre which swings to the right when pacing but moves to the left if a beat from the patient is sensed which inhibits the box from discharging. It should be noted that although the needle may swing to the right indicating pacing, this only means that the box has discharged and not necessarily that the stimulus has reached the heart (Figs. 5.7 and 5.8). A device can be fitted at the back of the pacing box to count the number of paced beats per hour.

The pacemaker box must be kept near the patient, either hanging on the bedhead or bedside or placed on a locker. There should be enough cable to allow free movement so that if the

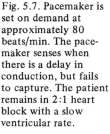

Fig. 5.7. Pacemaker is set on demand at approximately 80 beats/min. The pacemaker senses when there is a delay in conduction, but fails to capture. The patient remains in 2:1 heart block with a slow ventricular rate.

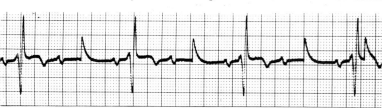

patient leans forward or turns over, the box is not dragged or the connections torn apart. For extra safety a wooden spatula or tongue depressor can be used as a splint supporting the junction box. Strap the pacing wire to the splint at one end and the pacemaker cable at the other, but avoid covering the screws. When a patient with a carrying box sits out of bed it is advisable to place the box on the floor rather than on the bed or stool as it can fall no further.

If he is able, the patient should realize his responsibilities towards caring for the equipment but he must not be allowed to tamper with the controls.

Once the pacemaker wire is proved to function correctly it can be attached directly on to a smaller pacing unit with no cable which is attached to the patient's upper arm with bandages or straps (Fig. 5.9). It can be held in place by elastic netting, such as 'netelast', which is strapped at the top and bottom to prevent the box from slipping. Controls should be accessible through the holes in netting and connections left free to be checked regularly. This system is best used immediately for confused patients to lessen the risk of the box falling to the floor.

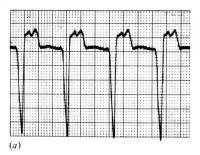

(a)

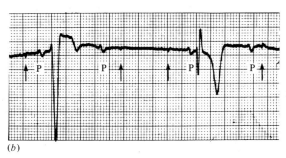

(b)

Fig. 5.8. (a) Pacemaker set at 90 beats/min. (b) Pacemaker then fails to capture so rhythm reverts to complete heart block. The pacing artefacts (↑), showing that the box is still functioning, are tiny and could be missed if there is excessive somatic tremor, or confused with p wave (P).

Fig. 5.9. (*a*) Meditek demand pacemaker box for temporary use. The pacing wire can be connected directly into the box but access is easier if a junction box is used. Note that when it is not in use both dials are pushed as far anti-clockwise as possible to conserve the batteries as there is no on/off switch. The box can be attached to the patient's arm in a netelast bag. Keep the screwdriver nearby.

(*b*) Devices (demand or fixed) pacemaker box for temporary use. The pacemaker wire terminals plug into the top of the box where they are screwed tightly in place. Each control box is clearly labelled. The box can be strapped to the patient's arm using the holders on the sides. No screwdriver is needed with this model.

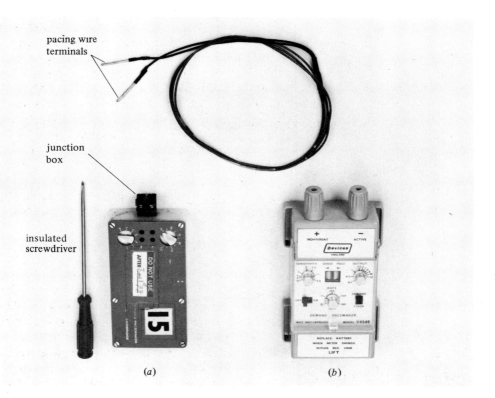

(*a*)   (*b*)

The screwdriver must be always accessible if it is needed for a particular type of box. Strap it to the bedhead or locker top. Most nurses on a Coronary Care Unit tend to carry an electrical (insulated) screwdriver. Another useful implement is a tool for cutting the plastic covering of the cable to expose more wire if it breaks. The wire can be quickly laid up and re-inserted.

If the entry site chosen is the right or left antecubital fossa there is great danger that the wire will slip out of the ventricle when the patient moves his arm. Therefore it is wise to splint the arm firmly to the patient's side, giving absolute immobility. As this is most uncomfortable for the patient for any length of time the site should not be used unless absolutely necessary. Although the entry is more dangerous and difficult initially the subclavian vein allows the patient most freedom of movement with least danger to the wire.

Insertion of temporary wire using an electrocardiogram
If no X-ray equipment is available the wire can be advanced in an emergency from a vein into the right ventricle safely using a 12 lead ECG machine, preferably a battery-operated model. Connect the limb electrodes of the machine to the patient. The V lead is connected to the distal terminal of the pacing electrode which acts as an exploring electrode transmitting activity to the machine where it is written out. The second pacing wire terminal may be attached to the positive input on the pacemaker box. As the electrode tip passes into the atrium a large negative P wave appears. When the right ventricle is reached the P wave becomes smaller but the QRS complex enlarges. The wire is then moved about gently until a satisfactory position is found, with a reasonable threshold. ST segment elevation occurs when the electrode contacts the myocardium.

Inserting a temporary wire in an emergency
A large spinal needle may be inserted directly into the left ventricle anteriorally between fourth and fifth or fifth and sixth ribs. The stylet is withdrawn and the pacing electrode passed into the needle and advanced until contact is made with the endocardium. The needle is then withdrawn leaving the pacing wire in place which is attached to a pacing box and stitched. Complications can occur such as trauma to the coronary arteries, pericardial tamponade, and there is more danger of dysrhythmias as the ventricu-

lar muscle is invaded. Once the emergency is over a second temporary wire can be sited in a more conventional place.

If a unipolar wire is inserted (i.e. one electrode at the tip) it must be connected to an indifferent electrode to function as a pacemaker. This is achieved by strapping a metal electrode plate on to the skin to which the positive terminal of the pacemaker is attached by a short length of wire. The negative terminal of the pacemaker box is connected to the pacing wire. A needle may be used as the distant electrode but if the patient is conscious it may be uncomfortable as it emits a tingling sensation.

Complications
Care must be taken to protect the patient from further problems as a result of pacing. Complications include the following.
(1) Infection — during the pacing procedure; or secondary infection at the site of entry of the wire.
(2) Haematoma at the site of entry. This can become so large that the trachea is obstructed, if the wire enters the internal jugular vein or subclavian vein, particularly if it is bilateral.
(3) Excess pain. The procedure is sometimes a little uncomfortable but if the site is very sore a different area may be better (e.g. if the subclavian route is chosen the wire may press against the bone).
(4) Wire lodging in coronary sinus or inferior vena cava. If this is a persistent problem a less malleable wire may allow more control.
(5) Damage to tricuspid valve.
(6) Perforated septum or ventricle. This occasionally occurs while pacing a patient with a fresh myocardial infarction.
(7) Pneumothorax. The lung may be punctured if the introducing needle slips out of a vein in the neck, causing an apical pneumothorax. A routine chest X-ray following the procedure will demonstrate this as well as confirming and recording the position of the wire. If pneumothorax has occurred the patient must remain sitting up until it is resolved or a chest drain is inserted.
(8) Ventricular fibrillation. This may be directly due to irritation by the wire or as a result of the dysrhythmia for which the pacemaker is inserted. The patient's rhythm should be observed for malfunction in the pacemaker box or wire.
(9) Secondary dysrhythmias caused by the pacing wire. (*a*) If the tip of the wire is not in good electrical contact with the epi-

cardium there may be insufficient voltage to stimulate the myocardium so that the patient's slow rhythm continues. This may be remedied by increasing the voltage on the box or by re-positioning the wire. (*b*) The tip may embed itself in a necrosed area of the myocardium, post-infarct. Although the myocardium contracts the small local intracardiac ECG is not received by the pacing box. It is not inhibited and acts like a fixed rate pacemaker (Fig. 5.10). This can be dangerous if the stimulus occurs on the T wave of a beat, causing ventricular tachycardia or fibrillation.

Care of the patient after insertion of a temporary pacing wire
Once the wire is stitched in place the patient may be sat up, particularly if he is dyspnoeic. Normally the wire should be firmly strapped in place first. The occlusive dressing should be checked for bleeding shortly afterwards, then routinely, and changed when necessary. Daily dressing should be avoided as it increases the risk of dislodging the wire as well as the possibility of introducing infection. The patient must not be allowed to wet the area.

The threshold should be checked daily following the procedure used during insertion. If it increases by a large amount (i.e. more than 0.5 V) in a day the doctor should be informed. It will be marginally higher on the second day as inflammation occurs around the tip of the wire, increasing the resistance.

A daily temperature check is essential and signs of fever reported. Septicaemia is an uncommon but unpleasant hazard. If there is evidence of inflammation the wire should be removed and sent for culture.

Nurses and doctors alike should be in the habit of looking at the connections whenever they are near the patient (Fig. 5.11).

A daily check of electrolytes prevents the possibility of imbalance altering the susceptibility of the myocardium to excitation by the wire with the risk of rhythm disturbance.

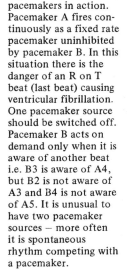

Fig. 5.10. There are two pacemakers in action. Pacemaker A fires continuously as a fixed rate pacemaker uninhibited by pacemaker B. In this situation there is the danger of an R on T beat (last beat) causing ventricular fibrillation. One pacemaker source should be switched off. Pacemaker B acts on demand only when it is aware of another beat i.e. B3 is aware of A4, but B2 is not aware of A3 and B4 is not aware of A5. It is unusual to have two pacemaker sources − more often it is spontaneous rhythm competing with a pacemaker.

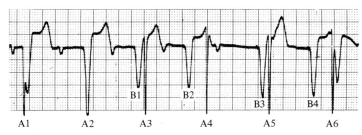

If a daily 12 lead ECG is helpful in the general care of the patient, such as after a myocardial infarction, then it is preferable to record the patient's own rhythm. Daily paced ECGs are not of interest. When switching off a pacemaker box for any reason it should never be done suddenly. Turn the rate control down slowly to allow the patient's spontaneous rhythm to develop. If the box is immediately switched off asystole may occur. If there is continuous pacing at a rate of 50 beats/min it is unsafe to lower the rate further as dangerous escape rhythms may occur, such as ventricular tachycardia.

Re-positioning a wire

If, within hours of the initial insertion of a temporary pacing wire, the position is found to be unsatisfactory, the skin stitch can be cut and the wire moved about until a better place is found. Sterility should be observed. Prophylactic antibiotic cover is sometimes prescribed as the site of entry is disturbed.

If the wire is to be re-positioned later the doctor judges whether to introduce a new wire at a different site rather than risk introducing infection from the protruding end of the wire. A fresh site will be necessary if the wire is removed because of infection.

Removal of a temporary wire

When it is considered that the patient no longer needs a pacemaker the box is switched off and the wire withdrawn. If there is doubt, e.g. after a myocardial infarction when the area of damage may extend thus jeopardizing the conducting system, the wire may be left *in situ* with the box switched off but set ready for immediate use. Sometimes the wire is left *in situ* and the box

Fig. 5.11. Drawing to illustrate where accidental disconnections may occur while a temporary pacemaker is in use. * marks areas where accidental disconnections occur. 1. The screw-in knobs may loosen so the hooks on the patient cable become detached. The push-in variety may easily pull out if they are loose. Check regularly that they are tight. 2. Wires detach from the hook. 3. Cable wires detach from junction box – check both before the pacing wire is inserted by tugging firmly at the connections. If only a few strands of wire are holding them together they will come apart. 4. Electrode wire falls out of junction box. Check this when the wire is connected at the junction box and at regular intervals by pulling the electrode terminals to ensure they do not slip out. If a wire breaks off, perhaps through an accident, while the pacing box is in use, remove about half an inch of plastic covering the wire to quickly reconnect it to continue pacing. Wire strippers are an asset in a ward where pacemakers are commonly in use, cf. Fig. 5.1.

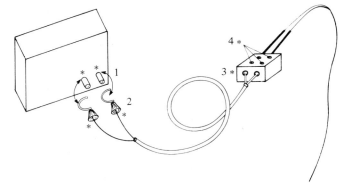

detached. Special care must be taken to insulate the terminals thoroughly by covering them separately in rubber. Before removing the wire the skin stitch is cut and a small gauze pad prepared. As the wire is withdrawn, gently to prevent cardiac irritability, a pressure pad is strapped over the area and left for several hours. A smaller plaster can then be used for a few days to cover the puncture and minimize the chance of infection.

When removing a single wire it can be done 'blind', i.e. without X-ray equipment. This is so when removing the temporary wire after the patient has an epicardial unit implanted. However, when the patient has an endocardial unit, care must be taken not to dislodge the permanent wire so it is important to withdraw the temporary wire while using an image intensifier to screen both wires.

Some pacemaker wires are disposable but most can be used again. They are expensive, so, if a wire is to be removed in a general ward or when a patient dies, the staff should realize that the wire must not be cut or thrown away. Having cleaned the wire and checked that it is intact it is soaked in cidex for three hours. It should not be allowed to soak for too long, otherwise it will begin to disintegrate. γ-radiation is more usually used for sterilization.

Permanent pacing

Long-term pacing can be achieved by placing a battery operated pacemaker box in the chest wall or abdomen with an electrode wire in contact with the endocardium or fixed to the epicardium. This is useful for patients with:

(1) residual dysrhythmias following myocardial infarction such as complete heart block or combinations of bundle branch block;

(2) fibrosis of the conduction system resulting in complete heart block (with or without Adams Stokes' episodes), intermittent bundle branch block with Adams Stokes' episodes, or sick sinus syndrome;

(3) congenital dysrhythmias such as bradycardia or tachydysrhythmias, or both these problems known as the brady/tachy syndrome.

Age should not be an impediment to implanting a pacemaker. A 98-year-old gentleman had the problem of falling off his bicycle as he cycled to his allotment because his heart rate was too slow. A pacemaker soon restored him to full activity. If an elderly patient has had a slow rhythm for a number of months or years there may be some mental impairment but, by implanting a pacemaker, amazing recovery can occur. A doubly incontinent, uncommunicative lady can become a normal sociable person again.

Before inserting a permanent pacemaker unit the type of power used is considered. Mallory cells are in common use. These are zinc mercuric oxide battery cells, providing a total output of 6 V. However, these last only 18 months to three years, when the patient has to undergo another operation to change the box. If local anaesthesia is used it is not too troublesome and many elderly people are given this type of unit.

Nuclear pacemakers were thought to be a possibility as this power source is capable of a long life, but radiation hazards exist if the box is damaged or destroyed in an accident and, when the patient dies, the box has to be dealt with.

Various types of lithium battery-operated pacemaker are now in common use as they last for four to twenty years, so are useful for younger people.

There are three basic methods used for implanting a permanent unit: transvenous, transthoracic or transmediastinal. Transvenous is the most common approach. Local anaesthesia only is needed. An incision is made over a vein in the neck or subclavicular area where the pacing wire enters. It is advanced until the tip reaches the apex of the right ventricle where protrusions attached near the tip burrow amongst the papillary muscle or trabeculae carneae. Other wires are plain with a radio-opaque line and rely on good initial positioning to keep them in place. Then the proximal end of the wire is directed downwards through the tissue to reach the pacemaker box which is placed in a pocket made in the chest wall on the same side as the wire enters. Care is taken in positioning it so that not too large a bump shows, both for comfort and cosmetic reasons. Special consideration is given for people with particular activities, such as 'cello playing, so that sets of muscles are not impeded.

Transthoracic entry is performed under general anaesthetic since the chest is opened anterolaterally between the fifth and sixth ribs to expose the left ventricle. Pacing electrodes are sutured directly on to the outer wall of the ventricle or screwed into it, before the wire is pushed through tissue to the abdominal wall where it is connected to the pacemaker box. Chest drains are left *in situ* post-operatively.

Transmediastinal insertion does not necessitate opening the pleural cavity so no chest drains are needed. The electrodes are sewn to the right ventricle.

If local anaesthesia only is needed the length of stay in hospital is less and morbidity is reduced. Many elderly patients, in need of a permanent device, are unfit for a general anaesthetic or fearful of it.

Babies or young people need an extra length of pacing wire to allow for growing so the transthoracic approach is used so that extra wire can be coiled in the abdomen.

Complications
Similar complications exist as for temporary pacing (p. 86) with a few additions.

(1) Diaphragmatic stimulation is sometimes a problem which can be very uncomfortable and may necessitate resiting the wire.

(2) Pericardial inflammation is possible if epicardial electrodes are used.

(3) Necrosis of the skin overlying the pacemaker box or wire can occur if the skin is drawn too tightly across it. If the box or wire erodes through it will need replacing. Rejection problems do not occur as the material in which the circuit is embedded is silicone rubber which is compatible with body tissue.

(4) Pacing may be interrupted for several reasons. The box may function well but problems may develop with the wire. The electrode may fracture if it is positioned awkwardly and is subject to constant stress. Inflammatory cells at the tip of the wire may occur so that the current cannot pass through the resistance, so there is no myocardial stimulation. The wire may erode through the vein and skin. Fibrosis of the endocardium or epicardium may fail to conduct the stimulation to the remaining myocardium thus insulating the heart from the electrical source, resulting in ineffective pacing (Fig. 5.10).

(5) Pacing stimulation may be inhibited by other muscular activity such as during coughing or sneezing. A different site for the box may improve matters.

(6) The pacemaker unit may fail. Premature battery failure accounts for a large number of pacing problems. This is usually predicted by a reduction in pulse rate when the voltage output is decreased so it sometimes fails to capture and occasionally there is a total absence of stimuli (Figs. 5.4 and 5.8).

Other problems include continuous discharge or, rarely, a runaway situation when the pacemaker discharges at a very rapid rate which may result in ventricular fibrillation.

Post-operative care following implantation of a permanent unit
To prevent physical complications, limb and chest exercises are encouraged and early mobilization is essential, especially for the elderly, to prevent such complications as retention of urine. The patient needs a balanced diet with plenty of fresh food, and a good fluid intake. Initial observation for rhythm disturbances is essential.

Discharge home. Once a patient is ready for discharge home he will be more confident about his pacemaker. Many questions will have been answered before the implantation as a doctor will explain fully, in most cases, the implications prior to gaining consent for the operation. Some patients are so ill before pacing that they will have no knowledge of the procedure so explanations are given when health is restored.

Specific instructions are needed about activity and he must be made aware of other hazards. The information given should be geared to his intellectual level. All electrical equipment which he uses must be properly grounded, e.g. electric razor, lawn mower. Some electrical apparatus produces high frequency signals which can inhibit a demand pacemaker. This includes diathermy and electrocautery equipment so the patient should always tell a doctor, dentist or other medical practitioner that he has a pacemaker. When passing through customs control the electronic eye must be avoided which may compete with the pacemaker. It is advisable for the patient to carry a card giving details about his box.

Although it is important that the patient does not become over-anxious about his pacemaker he should realize the importance of reporting specific symptoms such as dizziness, syncopal episodes, hiccoughs, palpitations, slowing heart rate, pain and breathlessness. He should feel his pulse regularly and understand the reason for a change in rate.

The importance of attending follow-up clinics regularly must be impressed upon him or a close friend or relative.

Before discharge various parameters are checked and recorded for comparison at later visits. These include:
(i)   a 12 lead ECG;

(ii)   anterior and lateral chest X-rays;

(iii) current delivered by the pacemaker;

(iv)   pacing artefact size;

(v)   threshold, if possible;

(vi)   rate — a magnet placed over the pacing box will cause it to pace in the fixed mode and will be measurable despite any natural rhythm.

(vii) P to QRS interval if a synchronized or sequential unit is used;

(viii) the escape interval is measured, i.e. the time taken for a paced beat to occur after a spontaneous beat.

The date of operation, any problems encountered and the type of pacemaker box is also recorded.

Follow-up care. The pacemaker is usually checked routinely two days after insertion to ensure satisfactory function. If there are no complications the patient may be discharged home, if he lives locally, but asked to return for removal of stitches in six to ten days. The patient is usually discharged after the stitches are removed.

The first out-patient check is normally one month after the operation. The patient is asked about his general health, his attitude to the pacemaker is discussed, and he is examined for signs of infection at the site of entry of the wire or over the stitch line.

The function of the pacemaker is studied by comparing the parameters obtained at the initial check. An analyser is used which is attached to the patient like the limb leads of a 12 lead ECG. It measures pulse width, impulse intervals and studies the vectors (direction of current flow within the heart) in limb leads I, II and III.

The patient also has the opportunity, while attending the clinic, to speak to other patients with pacemakers.

Follow-up schedules are very variable. One following schedule might be at six-monthly intervals for a year, then annually for those patients with lithium iodide units. Six-monthly visits continue for patients with Mallory cells.

Patients who live at some distance from a hospital are sometimes given a pocket-sized pulse analyser. It simply measures the impulse interval in milliseconds and displays the result in digital form. He telephones the clinic weekly to report the figures which should not normally exceed a particular value. When the numbers increase admission is planned to change the unit.

Types of pacing

There are various pacemakers in use with circuitry designed for different functions. The pacing electrodes are made for individual boxes although they are mostly interchangeable.

Functions include:

Atrial pacing (Fig. 5.12)

This is sometimes considered as a temporary or permanent measure for treating bradycardias when the patient has good atrio-ventricular conduction with no atrial fibrillation or flutter. The advantages are that atrial transport function is preserved and there is less danger of ventricular competition. There are problems in maintaining a good pacing position, however.

Atrio-ventricular sequential pacing (Fig. 5.13)

This method simulates normal electrical events in the heart by pacing the atria, then, after a pre-set delay, the ventricle is paced. The pause is adjustable — different units have different values. This is useful when the cardiac function is impaired, resulting in hypotension, as it helps to restore the cardiac output with the aid of atrial transport function or atrial boost.

If the patient's atrial rate is greater than the rate set on the box the pacemaker will be inhibited. If the patient's atrial rate is slower but the ventricular rate is greater the pacemaker will stimulate the atria but not the ventricles. The pacemaker will be inhibited if both the atria and ventricles beat faster than the set

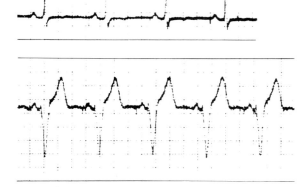

Fig. 5.12. Atrial pacing. Note small pacing artefact prior to each P wave.

Fig. 5.13. Atrio-ventricular sequential pacing.

rates but it will stimulate both if neither are as fast as the rate set on the box.

A wire for temporary use is available with four electrodes for atrial pacing and two electrodes for ventricular pacing. This has six terminals so special care must be taken to insulate those that are not in use. Fingers cut from a rubber glove and secured over the loose terminals are effective. The wire is inserted as if for normal ventricular pacing, then pairs of electrodes are tested. The pair with the lowest threshold is selected and connected to the pacing box.

Atrial synchronous ventricular pacing

A pacing wire with a separate electrode in the atria and ventricle is attached to a box having an atrial sensing circuit and a ventricular stimulating circuit. Having sensed atrial activity there is a preset delay before the ventricles are stimulated thus mimicking the PR interval. This system allows the atria to vary the ventricular rate for varying physiological demands (Fig. 5.14).

If atrial systole occurs the ventricles are automatically stimulated. If the atrial rate is excessive, such as in atrial tachycardia, the box simulates a 2:1 block or greater block to provide a reasonable cardiac rate.

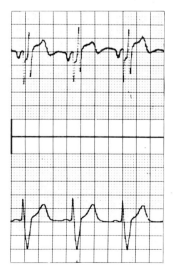

Fig. 5.14. Synchronous atrial pacing.

Rapid pacing

This is a temporary measure used to interrupt paroxysmal supra-ventricular or ventricular tachycardia. The pacemaker produces rapid stimulation until the tachycardia is interrupted and the patient's spontaneous rhythm takes over when pacing is discontinued.

These pacemakers are designed for special rhythm problems so the patient must become very intimate with the workings of the device so that it can be used to its full potential.

Further reading

Principles and techniques of cardiac pacing. S. Furman & D.J.W. Escher. New York; Harper & Row (1970).

Cardiac pacing, ed. Philip Samet & Nahil El-Sherif. New York; Grune & Stratton (1980).

Cardiac pacing – a concise guide to clinical practice. Philip Varriale & Emil A. Nacleiro. Philadelphia; Lea & Febiger (1979).

6. Pressure monitoring

Most patients admitted to a Coronary Care Unit need minimal pressure monitoring, particularly after the first few hours. Initially systolic and diastolic blood pressures are recorded regularly, such as every 15 minutes by conventional means, using a sphygmomanometer. Central venous pressure may be measured simply by means of an intravenous catheter and manometer which can be supplied from an intravenous bottle. An intravenous line is usually set up routinely in a patient admitted to a Coronary Care Unit.

However, some patients are admitted in a low output state, perhaps already in cardiogenic shock (systolic blood pressure below 80 mm Hg), when readings by conventional means are inadequate as they are inaccurate and are not continuous.

Other patients, such as those with a large infarct, with a history of previous infarcts or with persistent dysrhythmias, may be predicted to become more severely ill, so early pressure monitoring is useful and could help to prevent a state of collapse.

It is easier to insert intravenous lines when there is a reasonable pressure rather than attempting to cannulate a collapsed vein, which may then only be achieved by cut-down procedure which is time-consuming and more traumatic.

The heart consists of four chambers: right and left atria, right and left ventricles. The atria are thin-walled chambers into which blood flows at low pressure from the veins. Blood at high pressure leaves the right ventricle by the pulmonary artery through the pulmonary valve, and left ventricle by the aorta through the aortic valve. The tricuspid valve separates the atrium from the ventricle on the right side and the mitral valve on the left. Normally the atria beat together just before the ventricles beat synchronously.

The amount of blood the normal heart pumps over a given interval and the pressure needed to do this adequately are known, and these measurements are of prime importance to help physicians and surgeons assess the cardiac state of a patient. Circulation depends on blood being pumped out of the heart under pressure so that it flows towards a region of lower pressure. As the vascular system is a closed loop a change in one part of the system will affect other parts. The ventricles which pump the blood to the pulmonary system and systemic circulation are sensitive to their filling pressure so any pressure changes, particularly on the venous side of the heart, alter the ventricular performance. A simple example of this is haemorrhage where the venous blood returns to the right atrium at very low pressure and therefore the ventricular output is very low, so the blood pressure falls.

Individual chambers of the heart may fail due to congenital abnormalities, or damage from infarction or aneurysm. The valves may leak, causing stress to the heart. Systemic or pulmonary problems can affect the efficient working of the heart.

Many of the following conditions may be seen on a Coronary Care Unit secondary to coronary artery disease or as a result of a dysrhythmia.

Left heart failure
Primary left ventricular failure:
   coronary artery disease
   myocarditis (inflammation of cardiac muscle)
   cardiomyopathy (generalized degenerative disease of the
   heart)
Systolic overload of left ventricle:
   hypertension
   aortic valve disease.
Diastolic overload of left ventricle:
   mitral and aortic incompetence.
Systolic and diastolic overload of left ventricle:
   aortic stenosis and incompetence
   aortic stenosis and mitral incompetence.
Left atrial failure:
   mitral stenosis.

Right heart failure is usually secondary to left heart failure and is then called congestive cardiac failure. Pulmonary hypertension secondary to left heart failure causes back pressure on the right side of the heart, hence failure.

In health the average man pumps through each side of his heart about five litres of blood each minute. If the heart rate is 70 beats/min the heart will pump out about 70 ml blood at each heart beat to the lungs and body. This is called the stroke volume.

Starling's Law states that 'Stroke volume is dependent on the length of the muscle fibres prior to contraction. Thus the more distended the ventricles, the greater the stroke volume. The distension of the ventricles is in turn dependent on the venous return and effective venous filling pressure'.

The efficiency of the heart's pumping action largely depends on the cardiac muscle, the valves, the blood return to the heart and the resistance met by the blood forced out of the heart.

Peripheral resistance refers to the effect exerted mainly by the arterioles but also by the capillaries. The arterioles are maintained in a state of partial contraction called tone. They can be made to contract or relax in response to stimuli from the autonomic nervous system and circulating chemicals. It is this function of the arterioles which helps to keep the blood pressure in balance. Most capillaries are normally closed, and open to give a greater area for the blood to circulate and therefore decrease peripheral resistance. This in turn lowers blood pressure. Viscosity of blood contributes to peripheral resistance.

When the heart is working inefficiently, such as after a large myocardial infarction, sometimes the least resistance offered the better, so that greater blood flow is achieved to allow tissue perfusion. This may be done deliberately by using drugs which have a vasodilatory effect, thus increasing blood flow and therefore allowing greater oxygenation of the peripheral tissues.

The work done by the heart is determined by the cardiac output and the arterial resistance. Arterial resistance is sometimes called the *after load* and refers to the tension exerted by the walls of the artery during diastole.

There are some other phrases often used which may need further explanation.

Pre-load. The pressure at which blood returns to the heart.
End diastolic pressure (EDP) refers to the pressure in artery or chamber immediately prior to systole, so the vessel is in a 'resting' state. This may be pulmonary artery end diastolic pressure or left ventricular end diastolic pressure.
End diastolic volume. The volume in the ventricles immediately before contraction.
Mean. The average pressure for the total duration of the cycle.
Transducer. A device that converts mechanical power, e.g. pressure, into electrical power, e.g. waves on an oscilloscope, or vice versa.
Haematocrit. The relative volume of the cells to that of the blood — normally about 45%.
Viscosity. Stickiness, 'treacle-like' quality.

There are various methods for measuring cardiac output and other related functions of the heart such as stroke volume, cardiac work, pulmonary and arterial pressures and peripheral resistance. Simple inexpensive equipment is available or more expensive and complicated electronic devices. The sort of information which is helpful in treating the patient is decided, then the appropriate available equipment considered for use.

If central venous pressure alone is required, then a simple catheter with a saline manometer can be set up, but if the patient needs thorough pressure monitoring a more complicated type of catheter attached to electronic apparatus can perform several more functions, such as measuring pulmonary artery pressure and cardiac output.

Instruments function in different ways, so complications of measuring particular parameters should be considered. Frequent blood sampling may be an essential prerequisite for a particular instrument to perform, which will reduce haematocrit and therefore may be inadvisable for some patients. There may be problems in ensuring accuracy of the instrument, e.g. calibration must be constant and may require the attendance of an electronics technician.

Other instruments save the patient a lot of discomfort, such as relieving the need for frequent arterial punctures with risks of damage to the vessel, haemorrhage and infection. More rest may be allowed as the blood pressure readings are taken continuously by the instrument. He may also be made less anxious as he is disturbed less often when remote measuring devices are used.

Other factors that need to be considered when deciding to monitor a patient include: (a) ease of setting up the measuring instrument, particularly in an emergency; (b) availability of instruments in a low care and high care area; (c) expertise of nurses who will be left to care for the patient linked to such devices.

Various types of catheters are available for different purposes, so the doctor considers what parameters he would like to measure, for how long and if there is any added risk of damage to a vessel during insertion, use and removal of the catheter.

All catheters (i.e. intraluminal probes) are affected by movement within the vessel caused by blood flow or turbulence, or patient movement if placed in a vulnerable area. Artefacts may be superimposed on the trace, distorting readings. There is risk of infection and haemorrhage at the site of entry. However, catheters may be inserted peripherally and advanced to almost any part of the cardiovascular system. One catheter may perform several tasks, such as infusing fluids and drugs, measuring central venous pressure (CVP), pulmonary artery pressure and cardiac output.

Simple devices such as a saline manometer, graduated scale and spirit level for reading CVP are less likely to go wrong than complicated electronics, but the system is arguably less accurate. It does not offer a continuous reading, however, which is instantly available with electronic instruments.

Conditions that require particularly close haemodynamic observations are:
(1) low cardiac output state, e.g. cardiogenic shock, hypovolaemia;
(2) prior to, during or following major surgery, particularly cardiac;
(3) trauma, e.g. road traffic accident, severe burns.

Many parameters may be measured in conjunction for constant assessment. These include:
heart rate
heart rhythm
central venous pressure
atrial pressure
pulmonary artery pressure
pulmonary artery wedge pressure
systemic arterial pressure (systolic and diastolic)
cardiac output
urinary output
peripheral and core temperature.

Electronic instruments

Disadvantages	Advantages
Expensive to buy	Accurate
Expensive to run	Faster response to change
Need expert (technician) available in case of failure	Continuous display of readings
Difficult to sterilize	Several readings available from one or two catheters linked to one instrument
Electrical hazard	
There are more parts to fail	May often be linked to more than one patient

This necessitates attaching several lines to the patient for measuring and recording purposes. Equipment for assessing *heart rate* and *rhythm* have been dealt with in Chapters 2 and 3.

Central venous pressure (CVP)

This gives guidance to the body's state of hydration. A central line may also be set up for infusing particular drugs and for parenteral feeding. CVP is measured in the right atrium or superior vena cava in the intra-thoracic cavity. Venous blood returning to the right side of the heart normally flows at a low pressure (0—6 mm Hg) into the superior vena cava and right atrium. This pressure may be raised above normal values when the intra-thoracic pressure (normally below atmospheric pressure) is increased, such as during intermittent positive pressure ventilation. Other conditions which raise right-sided pressure are constrictive pericarditis, cardiac tamponade, pulmonary oedema, hypervolaemia and cardiogenic shock. Hypovolaemia lowers central venous pressure.

CVP is only a guide to left atrial pressure but if a normal pressure is established which then rises without other obvious causes it suggests impending pulmonary oedema. Pulmonary oedema is likely to occur at about 24 mm Hg, but often not until the pressure is 30 mm Hg or higher.

Equipment for measuring CVP

> A radio-opaque i.v. catheter which will reach from the site of entry so that the tip settles in the superior vena cava or right atrium
>
> Giving set
>
> Manometer (attached at one end to the giving set and at the other to the i.v. catheter)
>
> i.v. fluid — normally sodium chloride 0.9%; dextrose may be used
>
> Scale
>
> Sighting device or spirit level, or pressure transducer attached to a recording instrument.

Method

The vein to be entered is chosen. Typically the median cubital or basilic vein in the ante-cubital fossa, the subclavian vein, or the internal jugular vein are used. The internal jugular is often used as there is less danger of accidental displacement of the cannula or excess movement with the possibility of infection or haemorrhage as the patient moves and it is less inhibiting for him. The procedure using this route takes less time.

If an arm vein is used it is advisable to immobilize the arm with a splint. The chosen area is shaved if necessary and cleansed. The i.v. and manometer lines are filled and manometer attached to the scale. Local anaesthetic is infiltrated into the area. An incision is made in the skin and the catheter introduced into the vein and advanced to a measured length to ensure that it reaches the superior vena cava or right atrium.

Site of the tip of the CVP line can be confirmed by using an ECG machine but this may constitute an electrical hazard (see Chapter 8), so a battery-operated instrument is best used. Fluoroscopy may be used while inserting the line to achieve a good position quickly.

Complications which may arise during insertion include: introduction of infection; haemorrhage; perforation of a vein; puncture in an artery; pneumothorax (if the subclavian vein is chosen); nerve damage; rarely cardiac tamponade; atrial dysrhythmias if the tip lies in the right atrium.

The manometer line is attached to the cannula and a reading is taken. If the tip lies within the intra-thoracic cavity the fluid in the column will rise and fall with respiration. Once in the optimum position it is sutured to the skin if it is to be left for any length of time, or strapped securely. A plain chest X-ray will confirm the position of the tip of the cannula but if it is not easily seen a small amount of radio-opaque dye can be injected immediately prior to X-ray.

The i.v. fluid is set to run very slowly, usually just enough to keep the line patent, particularly in cardiac patients whose sodium intake is kept to a minimum.

If a second line of fluid such as blood or plasma is attached to the CVP catheter via a three-way tap, it should be switched off and the saline allowed to run for a few moments to clear the length of the catheter each time before a reading is taken, to ensure accuracy.

Point of reference at which reading is taken
Opinions vary a little but the general aim is that the zero on the scale is level with the right atrium or where the tip of the catheter is calculated to be — verified on chest X-ray.

Reference points generally chosen are: (*a*) sternal notch; (*b*) sternal angle; (*c*) level of right atrium, calculated to be a point where a line drawn down from the mid axilla crosses a line level with the fourth intercostal space on the right chest wall (Fig. 6.1).

Whichever point is chosen, it is important that the reading is always taken with reference to the same place, so that point should be clearly marked with a skin pencil.

Taking a reading

Initially, readings are taken every 15 minutes, decreasing to half-hourly, then hourly when the patient's condition is more stable.

It is preferable that the patient lies flat on his back for every reading but this is usually impractical. Levelling the graduated column helps to keep the reading accurate if the patient is sitting up a little, but the reading will be much lower if he is sat upright for a particular reading, so this information should be noted on his chart.

Concessions are made, such as using the right atrial level while he is on his back and the sternal angle while on his side. Before moving a patient, consider if he is in a better position for a CVP reading before or afterwards, particularly as the apparatus is set up on one side of the bed and is difficult, if not impossible, to move.

Ensure that the catheter is free of blood or other plasma-expanding fluids. Switch off any other i.v. lines which may be attached, so that no pressure can be transmitted from them.

Fig. 6.1. Simple fluid manometer for measuring central venous pressure. The central mark on the scale is set to the level of the chosen reference point (here it is the mid-axillary line). The tap is turned to disconnect the scale from the infusion bottle and to connect it to the patient.

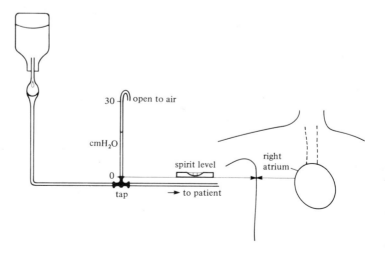

Ensure the saline infusion is running freely by turning it on quickly for a few seconds. If the infusion rate is sluggish, take steps to clear it.

Check that the zero on the scale is level with the mark on the patient's body, using the spirit level or sighting device. Using the three-way tap, run saline up the manometer column above the expected CVP level.

Turn the tap to allow the column of fluid to flow into the patient while watching it continuously. If it falls quickly air may enter the i.v. line on the patient's side of the three-way tap where it is difficult to remove quickly; there it is time-wasting and may risk air embolus if it is not noted.

When pressure levels equalize, fluid in the column will rise and fall about a figure on the scale due to respiration, normally between 0 and 7 cm water or 0 and 6 mm Hg.

Problems that may occur
No fall in the column. The i.v. line is probably blocked or kinked. Look for kinks, particularly where the line enters the patient as the weight of the line may bend if it is not firmly secured. It is helpful to take a loop in the line so that it is held in a bend which cannot kink. This loop also ensures that a tug on the line will not dislodge the catheter.
The level falls but there is no respiratory swing. This is usually due to displacement of the line outside the intra-thoracic cavity. Check the line at the site of entry or confirm by fluoroscopy or chest X-ray. To prevent the line slipping out it should be stitched *in situ* or strapped in such a way that it is very difficult to move. If a catheter has slipped out it should not be pushed back into the vein as this risks infection. A new line should be inserted.

When a patient is attached to a continuous CVP recording device the transducer should be kept level with the right atrium or other known convenient point. The transducer could be mounted on a perspex platform or attached to a part of the instrument. A levelling device, usually a spirit level, is used.

There is usually a continuous wave-form display. These readings should not be recorded as correct until proper levelling is ensured. Often there is provision for a write-out of the pressure waves, which may be recorded at 25 mm/s or 25 cm/h.

The instrument is calibrated to a known level which does not normally differ from day to day but should be checked each time when setting it up for use.

A device is added which automatically flushes regularly and can also be used manually.

Flattening of the trace. This may be due to blockage in the catheter, bubbles in the catheter or transducer. Therefore clear the line until the trace improves.

Trace disappears. Calibration needs adjusting, or position button may have been moved.

Dressing
Opinions vary about dressing the entry site. Some doctors prefer an occlusive dressing which is left alone so there is less risk of contamination and dislodgement, while others prefer the site to be looked at daily, followed by a dressing using aseptic technique.

Infusion of drugs
If a drug is infused, such as isoprenaline when a small regular dose is given continuously, it is better to set up a separate line so that the effects of the drug are not interrupted.

Atrial pressure recording following cardiac surgery
Catheters are introduced through the chest wall into the right and left atrium during operation. 5% dextrose is infused slowly through each. A three-way tap with a side arm is set up and the column of fluid supported by pressure exerted by the atrium is measured using the same reference point each time on the chest. The point represents the level of atria within the chest (Fig. 6.2).

Pulmonary artery pressure and pulmonary artery wedge pressure
Pulmonary artery pressure gives an indication of venous return to the left heart and right ventricular function.

Pulmonary wedge pressure gives a direct indication of left atrial pressure which approximates resting left ventricular pressure; therefore it can help to assess left ventricular function.

Equipment
Have the defibrillator at hand as the right ventricle is entered
A long radio-opaque catheter, often marked at 10 cm intervals,
    with an inflatable balloon at the tip
Cut-down set if used, or i.v. tray
Skin cleansing solution

Giving set
i.v. fluid, bag of 0.9% sodium chloride (500 ml with 500 units of
     heparin)
Pressure bag around bag of i.v. fluid pumped to 300 mm Hg
Pressure recording instrument
Pressure transducer
Flushing device such as an 'intraflow'
Pressure manometer tubing (200 cm length) to attach transducer
     to i.v. catheter
Two stopcocks
1 ml syringe

Procedure
Typically the vein in the right or left ante-cubital fossa is entered,
using a cut-down technique.
     When the tip of the i.v. catheter reaches the right atrium the
balloon is inflated to assist the movement into the right ventricle
and into the pulmonary artery where it wedges in a smaller
branch. The balloon is immediately deflated.

Fig. 6.2. Chest X-ray
showing position of
Swan Ganz pressure
line with the tip resting
in the left pulmonary
artery (arrow) for a
wedge pressure reading
to help assess left heart
function. The catheter
enters the subclavian
vein, passes into the
superior vena cava and
right atrium, through
the tricuspid valve into
the right ventricle,
through the pulmonary
valve and into the pul-
monary artery.

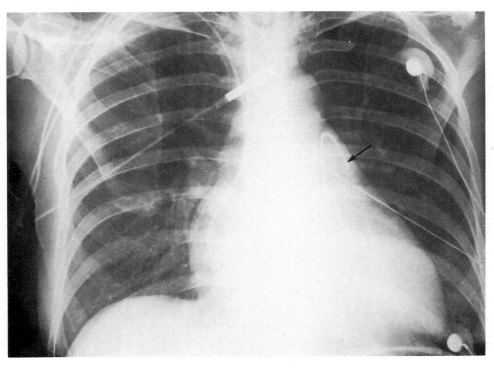

Fluoroscopy is often used to help site the catheter, or the pressure waves may be studied on the recording instrument.

Once in the optimum position the catheter is sutured in place or firmly strapped, and the site dressed.

Problems associated with pulmonary artery catheters
Introduction of infection
Haemorrhage at site of entry
Atrial and ventricular dysrhythmias
Pulmonary infarct if the balloon is left inflated.

The catheter is attached to the pressure manometer line which connects to the transducer. This is attached to the recording instrument via the flushing device.

Pulmonary artery pressure waves are displayed continuously on an oscilloscope and their value can be read against a scale at the side of the screen (Fig. 6.3). It can be difficult to calculate them accurately as allowance must be made for respiratory swing. The pressure wave on the oscilloscope can be compared with analogue or digital displays with averaging to give a true reading. Normal pulmonary artery systolic pressure is about 18 mm Hg (mean).

Wedge pressure is obtained by inflating the balloon with air or carbon dioxide so that the small pulmonary artery branch in which it sits is occluded. The pressure wave on the oscilloscope can be compared with the figures on the scale at the side of the screen, or read from analogue or digital display.

When originally inflating the balloon it should be noted how much air is needed and the same amount used each time to mini- mize the possibility of over-inflating it to cause damage to the vessel or to burst the balloon with the possibility of air or foreign body embolus. The usual amount is about 0.6 ml of air. The same 1 ml or 2 ml syringe can be used each time.

It is most important to deflate the balloon immediately after the reading to prevent infarction of the tissue beyond the balloon.

Prior to each reading the transducer should be level with a chosen point, usually the sternal notch, checked each time with a spirit level.

The instrument should be calibrated before it is set up and checked before taking the initial reading so there is a known zero level, then checked by a technician routinely daily or when a fault is suspected.

The entry site is usually inspected and dressed daily.

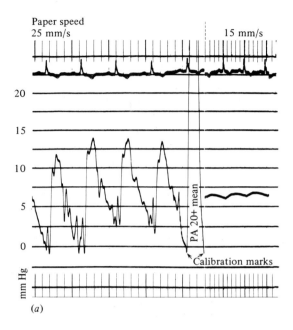

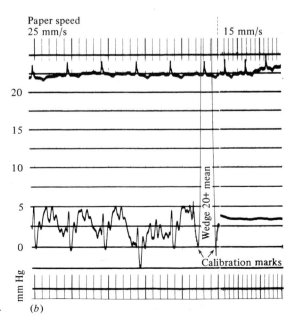

Fig. 6.3. Pulmonary artery pressure waves.

Problems that may occur after insertion. No pressure waves: line is clogged due to small lumen. Try to withdraw blood. If it comes easily, flush it several times to clear the line completely. If there is difficulty, try gentle flushing but do not force it. The i.v. catheter may have to be changed.

No wedge pressure: balloon has ruptured.

Ventricular ectopics: end of catheter may have slipped back into the right ventricle. It may float back into position if the balloon is inflated, but if it has slipped back at the site of entry it should not be pushed back in or there is a risk of introducing infection.

Flattening of waves: leak in three-way stopcock.

Change in wave form: catheter may have slipped marginally; check X-ray or fluoroscopy. Balloon was left partially inflated; deflate it. Catheter is beginning to clog; try flushing. Bubbles in the transducer dome; try flushing the line, having disconnected it from the patient first.

Drugs are not given routinely via the pulmonary artery line except in rare circumstances, so a second i.v. line is always set up for this purpose and for infusing fluids.

Blood samples are occasionally taken from the pulmonary artery line. Always ensure the line is thoroughly flushed afterwards.

Removal of central lines

Before removing a pulmonary artery line, atrial line or CVP line, consider if there are any other lines in proximity such as a pacing wire. Sometimes the lines twist around each other. If there is another line it is safer to remove the discontinued line using fluoroscopy (to prevent dislodgement of the remaining line) while a second person watches the cardiac monitor to warn of dysrhythmias.

Arterial pressure

Continuous assessment of systolic and diastolic pressure is achieved simply by insertion into a peripheral artery of an indwelling catheter which is attached to a pressure monitoring instrument (Fig. 6.4). The most convenient place to insert the catheter is the radial artery, although other peripheral arteries are occasionally chosen.

Equipment
Skin cleansing solution
Suture material (if used)
Short catheter
Pressure manometer line, usually 200 cm length
Pressure transducer
Infusion fluid in bag — normally 0.9% sodium chloride with
    Heparin (500 units per 500 ml fluid)
Pressure bag around infusion fluid pumped up to 300 mm Hg
Intraflow or similar flushing device
Stopcocks — 2
Recording instrument, ready calibrated

Method
The recording instrument is set up ready for use with the infusion
giving set attached to the transducer and pressure manometer
tubing connected to the patient side of the transducer. Run the
infusion fluid through the set, then, using the intraflow, fill the
manometer tubing.

The skin is shaved if necessary, cleansed and infiltrated with
local anaesthetic. The catheter is stabbed into the artery and
stitched or very firmly strapped in place.

Pressure is applied for a few moments and the site inspected
frequently, initially for signs of leakage and haematoma.

The manometer line is connected to the catheter.

On the recording instrument pressure waves should be seen
rising after each heart beat. There should be a clear wave-form so
that systolic and diastolic blood pressure can be compared with a

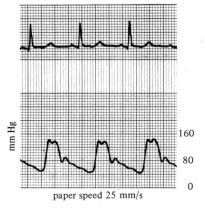

Fig. 6.4. Systemic
arterial pressure waves
with simultaneous
cardiac rhythm
recording.

mm Hg

160

80

0

paper speed 25 mm/s

scale at the side of the oscilloscope. If there is a second unused line on the oscilloscope this can be used as a reference line check as it can be quickly seen at a short distance. Choose a value which relates to the patient's pressure, such as 100 mm Hg if the patient's pressure is near that figure.

Analogue and digital displays ensure accurate interpretation and average out the figures over a few pressure cycles.

To ensure accuracy when the instrument is first set up, it is advisable to check the blood pressure reading, using a sphygmomanometer and stethoscope. Occasionally the wave-form signals 'overshoot', i.e. appear higher if there is insufficient 'damping' on the instrument.

There may be a dial on the instrument panel to alter the amount of damping. Over-damping produces a simplified trace which is unhelpful while studying pressure waves. Damping can be achieved also by deliberately introducing air bubbles into the system until an ideal trace is achieved. Conversely extraneous bubbles causing over-damping are flushed from the system (Fig. 6.5).

Very low pressure, which is difficult to detect normally, can be measured with an arterial line *in situ*. It is also worth checking the accuracy of using sphygmomanometer and stethoscope once the instrument is proved correct.

Care of the arterial line
Splint the limb if there is any possibility of the line becoming dislodged or kinked.

Manually flush the line at least hourly and observe it constantly for any signs of back flow.

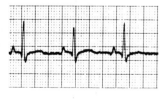

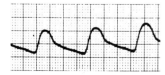

Fig. 6.5. Overdamped arterial pressure record. (See comparative trace, Fig. 6.4.)

Keep the pressure bag inflated to 300 mm Hg.

Never allow the flushing fluid bag to become empty.

Whenever blood samples are withdrawn from the line flush it until clear.

Problems that may arise
During insertion. (*a*) Introduction of infection (*b*) haemorrhage.
After insertion. (*a*) Secondary haemorrhage (when pressure increases): Have pressure bandage ready. (*b*) Ischaemia of limb distal to the artery. Report any signs of arterial occlusion: loss of pulses, mottled blue or pale skin, cold limb, numbness. The arterial line may need to be resited. Encourage the patient to move his fingers regularly. (*c*) Oedema of the hand or limb distal to arterial line. Raise the limb on a pillow and encourage the patient to exercise by clenching fists, or moving toes if an artery in the leg is used.
Problems on the oscilloscope. (*a*) Flattening of trace: line occluded with blood or blocked by air bubbles. Disconnect the line and flush it gently. (*b*) Loss of trace: patient has changed position of limb so catheter moves in relation to artery; splint it. Or line has come apart; splint and strap any suspect connections to ensure they do not accidentally come apart. The lumen of the catheter may be blocked by the vessel wall; saline can be flushed through easily but blood cannot be withdrawn as the wall acts as a non-return valve. Withdraw the catheter slightly.
Minor nuisances. These add to the problems of using pressure monitoring equipment.
(1) Leakage at the site of entry caused by: (*a*) Insecure connection, if it repeatedly comes apart change it; (*b*) insufficient immobility, use a splint if necessary, particular if the wrist or elbow is involved; (*c*) arterial line moves because there is insufficient strapping.
(2) Confusion of lines. Try not to allow any to cross the patient, so ensure the recording instrument is set up on the side where the catheter enters. Do not allow lines to cross over one another. Label them clearly if it is found helpful.
(3) Clotting in the line. Ensure the flushing system works efficiently; if not, change it. Manually flush once an hour and after each time that blood is withdrawn into the line.
(4) Bubbles of air in the line. Do not allow bubbles to enter the patient. Turn off the supply to the patient, then disconnect the tubing and flush it out. Never apply forced suction or

pressure to electronic transducers as the membrane may be damaged.

(5) Kinking of tubing. Ensure any loops or bends in the tubing do not impede the flow. Place a tension loop in the manometer and infusion lines to prevent them being disconnected.

(6) The position of the patient sometimes affects readings. If it is possible to replace the line, this is preferable, otherwise it should be noted how the best flow is obtained, e.g. holding the patient's head to one side, and ensure that all personnel receive this information.

Removal of the line

When it is decided to discontinue monitoring the arterial pressure, a manual blood pressure should be taken to ensure it is easily recordable. As the line is withdrawn a swab is held firmly against the puncture for at least five minutes, or longer if anticoagulant therapy is given. A pressure bandage is then applied and the distal part of the limb inspected regularly for signs of arterial occlusion, as a clot from the catheter site may be left in the artery.

Methods of measuring cardiac output

Cardiac output (output per ventricle per minute) = stroke volume (output per ventricle per beat) × heart rate (per minute).

Thermo-dilution

A catheter is introduced peripherally, which has an outlet in the right atrium and a temperature sensor, or thermistor, in the pulmonary artery.

A measured amount of cold saline at a known temperature is injected into the catheter, which mixes in the right atrium and flows into the pulmonary artery where the temperature of the blood/saline mixture is measured. The injected fluid is called coolant. Using tables relating to the measured temperature drop, blood flow through the right side of the heart is calculated.

Bolus doses of saline will give only intermittent readings, while continuous assessment is possible if there is a continual flow.

Dye dilution technique

Two catheters are required. One catheter is introduced into a peripheral vein so that the outlet lies near the heart, usually in the right atrium. The second catheter is introduced into an artery.

A known amount of indocyanine green dye, diluted in distilled water, is injected intravenously. The second catheter is attached to a motorized syringe which withdraws blood at a constant rate and allows it to pass through an instrument which measures its optical density so that the amount of dye can be found and, using tables, the cardiac output is calculated.

Using a computer that allows for recirculation of the dye, the cardiac output can be continuously assessed.

Another way of measuring blood flow is the ultrasonic flow metre which transmits ultrasonic sound waves to the blood in a blood vessel. It may be used in cuff, cannula or catheter tip form. Measurements of blood flow are determined either by timing sound carried by blood or by measuring the frequency shift of sound scattered from moving red cells. The latter is called the Doppler principle.

If a non-invasive technique is essential, ultrasound in cuff form is the only method.

Urinary output
In seriously ill patients when fluid balance is most important, a urinary catheter is usually used. A drainage container in which the urine can be accurately measured to the nearest cubic centimetre is essential.

The urine is usually measured hourly initially. A running balance is most helpful.

Peripheral and core temperature
A guide to good general perfusion is the colour, and temperature of the skin compared to core.

The most convenient and safest method is to place an indwelling thermistor probe in the rectum, attached to an electric thermometer. A second sensor is attached to a foot. The foot sensor can be used for both feet in turn. This is particularly important if one leg is at risk of interruption to blood flow, e.g. intra-aortic balloon *in situ*. Ensure the rectum is clear of faeces. Check at intervals that the probe and sensors are correctly in place.

Considerations about equipment
The preceding notes on monitoring pressure and blood flow emphasize accuracy, continuity of readings and least disturbance to the patient. This is only possible if good equipment is used: the best

that can be bought with the money available. The instruments are costly, and to use second-rate attachments is uneconomic. It is far more practical to use a high-quality stopcock which does not leak, fill with air or come apart, rather than to spend time coping with these problems, probably at the most inconvenient moment.

A great deal more work is being done in the field of pressure monitoring to improve on present-day methods. A quote from D.H. Bergel's book *Cardiovascular Fluid Dynamics*, Vol. 1, summarizes this neatly: 'The challenge is to remove from the measurement of pressure the need for both thought and skill.'

Further reading

The Human Heart − a guide to heart disease. Brendan Phibbs. New York; C.V. Mosby (1979).

Cardiovascular Fluid Dynamics, Ed. by D.H. Bergel, vols. 1 & 2. London & New York; Academic Press (1972). This is a series of papers on blood pressure and flow which cover the subjects in great detail.

An Introduction to Human Physiology. J.H. Green. Oxford Medical Publication (1974).

From Cardiac Catheterization Data to Hemodynamic Parameters. S.S. Yang, L.G. Bentivoglio, V. Maranhão & H. Goldberg. Philadelphia; F.A. Davis Company (1972).

7. Intra-aortic balloon pump

The intra-aortic balloon pump has been in use in many medical centres for a few years and has now become more widely available.

It is a mechanical system used to aid impaired circulation. Basically, an elongated balloon is introduced into an artery near the heart. It is inserted retrogradely through the femoral artery to lie in the descending aorta. Rarely the balloon is introduced antegradely into the ascending aorta through an intercostal incision. The balloon is attached to a power-operated gas pump.

At the beginning of diastole, when most of the coronary artery perfusion occurs, gas from a pressure pump inflates the balloon to increase aortic pressure. Blood in the aorta is displaced retrogradely, therefore pushing more blood into the coronary arteries. Blood is also pushed forward into the peripheral circulation. The balloon is then deflated by suction exerted by a vacuum as systole begins which lowers blood pressure in the aorta, thus reducing the work of the left ventricle. This is called counterpulsation. This extra boost can increase the circulation by up to five litres per minute (Fig. 7.1).

The pump can be timed to inflate the balloon during every diastolic period (1:1) or at lesser intervals of 1:2, 1:3, 1:4 or 1:8 depending on the machine used. As the patient's condition improves frequency can be decreased prior to stopping the pump. This is called 'weaning'.

Various conditions can be treated including the following.
(1) Ventricular aneurysm to increase blood pressure prior to and during surgical resection.
(2) Cardiogenic shock following myocardial infarction.

Fig. 7.1. Schematic diagram demonstrating the position of the intra aortic balloon in the descending aorta. (a) Balloon deflated; (b) Trisegmental balloon filling in the central portion first; (c) fully inflated balloon.

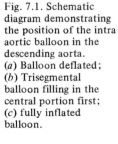
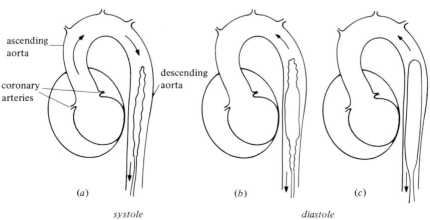

ascending aorta

coronary arteries

descending aorta

(a)   (b)   (c)

systole   *diastole*

(3) Shock caused by septicaemia.

(4) Ventricular septal rupture pre-operatively.

(5) Prophylactic support for other conditions requiring cardiac surgery, both pre- and post-operatively. Some patients requiring cardiac surgery can be improved to such an extent that surgical intervention is made possible whereas before it could not be considered.

(6) Following myocardial infarction to prevent the injured area from extending.

Benefits for the patient include: (a) increased myocardial and systemic perfusion; (b) less metabolic acidosis; (c) increased oxygen delivery; (d) improved renal perfusion.

The insertion of an aortic balloon pump allows the surgeon more time for further evaluation, and the patient's condition may become more stable, thus increasing his chance of survival after surgery. The surgeon can plan the operation more carefully and can arrange to have the best personnel and equipment available for optimum care during surgery and afterwards.

Equipment

Balloon

The balloon is made of very thin polyurethane polymer or similar material that is compatible with human tissue, with antithrombogenic properties. It is sterile, doubly wrapped, disposable and expensive. There is a radio-opaque line along its length and on the clear plastic tube which connects it to the source of gas.

Several sized balloons are available, from 10 cc for paediatric use to 40 cc for adults. 20, 30 and 40 cc balloons are commonly used. The size of the balloon used is usually decided by the size of the patient but it is not until the surgeon sees the dimension of the lumen of the aorta that he can really decide, so several sizes should be ready but wrapping should not be removed until the final decision is made. The largest size that will be accepted by the aorta is always used so that greatest efficiency is achieved.

The balloon may have one, two or three chambers, described as bi-directional, uni-directional and tri-segmental respectively. The tri-segmental balloon is most commonly used and has a central segment which inflates first, then the proximal and distal segments. This overcomes any tendency to trap blood in the aorta between the balloon and the wall of the aorta which may rupture with the increased pressure.

Gas

The gas used to inflate the balloon is either helium or carbon dioxide. These will be absorbed into the blood stream should a leak occur. A safety chamber prevents more than about 50 cc from escaping. The gas may be introduced from an outside source or, more safely, there is a limited amount in an enclosed system incorporated into the machine.

ECG monitoring

Electrodes for cardiac monitoring are attached to the pumping equipment. The electrodes are not disposable. They are made of high quality material to produce an optimum trace. They should be strapped securely in place over the trunk where there is least amount of skeletal muscle which may cause interference. When three electrodes are used it is recommended to position the right arm lead over the right clavicle and the left arm lead on the lower ribs on the left. The earth electrode can be placed anywhere convenient. This results in a trace similar to lead I or II on a 12 lead ECG. A five electrode system is sometimes employed so that any monitoring lead may be selected. To prevent the electrodes being dragged off, support the weight of the cable with a clip attached to the bedding, or patient's clothing.

As the ECG trace produced is used to trigger the gas pumping mechanism a high quality signal is essential for correct function and to give a minimal number of alarm states. Good skin preparation will help. It is the ventricular complex that triggers the machine to cause balloon deflation during systole and inflation during diastole so it must be clear and of a high enough amplitude to be detected by the machine. The configuration must be upright, i.e. an R wave so there is a switch on some models to change the polarity, i.e. reverse it.

Dysrhythmias should be suppressed as far as possible, although the very act of infusing an antidysrhythmic agent may decrease cardiac motility. Lignocaine is often used. Conversely, by increasing myocardial perfusion with the aid of the balloon pump, atrial and ventricular dysrhythmias are often suppressed. The mechanism can cope with tachydysrhythmias up to certain speeds (said to be approximately 200 beats/min) but, in practice, once the heart rate is above about 140 beats/min there are often difficulties.

The pump operates most efficiently when there is sinus rhythm at a rate between 70 and 100 beats/min.

Supraventricular tachycardia at a fast rate, such as paroxysmal atrial tachycardia, may not allow the balloon sufficient filling time, so the timing of inflation could be reduced to 2:1 to inflate during alternate periods of diastole.

Slow rates can be speeded up with the use of a pacemaker. If the heart rate is approximately the same as the pacemaker setting, they will compete to give some paced beats, some fusion (see Chapter 5) and some normal conduction. The changing configurations will confuse the balloon pump, so improved performance will be achieved by pacing at a higher rate or turning the demand paced unit down if the spontaneous rhythm is over 60 beats/min.

Before defibrillation the ECG cable should be disconnected from the balloon pump.

Preparation

Pump
Prior to inserting the balloon the machinery is set up ready for use. The workings of the intra-aortic balloon pump are housed in a mobile trolley. Different functions, controls and display panels are provided by manufacturers. The ECG signal is introduced and an arterial line, usually from the radial artery, is connected to give an arterial pressure trace. The ECG signal or pressure wave triggers the pump.

Patient
A consent form is signed by the patient or relative after explanation of the procedure and its aims.

The patient is shaved from umbilicus to upper thighs. He should lie on a radio-translucent bed so that fluoroscopy can be used during the insertion procedure, if needed, or to check the balloon's position later. Patient's observation charts, record sheets, notes and X-rays should be at hand.

General arrangement
If inserted in the open ward, a large enough area should be cleared to allow room for the surgeon to operate and for all the extra equipment. When choosing the site consider access to other patients. The area is screened and the bedhead moved away from the wall in case intubation and an anaesthetic machine or ventilator is needed. Intubation equipment and Ambubag with face-mask are prepared. Good lighting over the operating field is essential, so extra mobile theatre lamps may be used. Pacing equipment should be available for instant use if needed.

Nurse

The nurse who will care for the patient immediately after insertion should take the opportunity to assess the patient's general condition for herself — particularly his mental awareness and attitude and the condition of his lower limbs, e.g. presence or absence of popliteal and pedal pulses.

Insertion procedure

General anaesthetic may be used, particularly if it is inserted in theatre as part of the post-surgical care, but it is usually performed with local anaesthetic. Sterility is essential although it may be necessary to perform the operation in an open ward when the patient is too sick to move.

The arterial pulse is located, the skin cleansed and infiltrated with local anaesthetic prior to an incision using a scalpel blade. An opening is made in the artery. A dacron or teflon sleeve is slipped over the tubing of the balloon before it is inserted, balloon first, into the artery. When the optimum position is attained (by measuring the length of the balloon against the patient, or using fluoroscopy), the sleeve is sutured to the edges of the opening of the artery and the wound closed up.

Complications

These may be encountered during the insertion procedure, shortly afterwards or later.

(1) Difficulty in introducing the balloon into an artery. A change of site may be tried but atheroma is sometimes so extensive that introduction of a balloon proves impossible. Patients over 65 years are generally not considered for a balloon pump as atheroma is usually too advanced.

(2) Dissection of the aorta.

(3) Lifting atheromatous plaque to occlude the aorta.

(4) Haemorrhage at the site of entry.

(5) Haematoma.

(6) Impairment of circulation to the distal limb, causing numbness or, in extreme cases, gangrene. If circulation problems occur the patient is reassessed to consider if he will survive without the balloon, if immediate cardiac surgery is feasible or if the balloon must be re-sited on the other side.

Signs of circulatory impairment in the leg may be apparent during the insertion procedure or fairly soon afterwards. The patient complains of pain or numbness or pins and needles, impaired sensation and impaired movement. The leg becomes pale and cool, and popliteal, posterior tibial and dorsalis pedis pulses are now absent.

(7) Impairment of circulation in the renal arteries if the balloon is improperly sited.

(8) Introduction of infection.

(9) Thrombocytopenia.

Post-operative care

An X-ray is taken to confirm and record the position of the balloon pump.

Special attention is paid to:

(1) observation of wound for leakage: a pressure pad may be needed temporarily

(2) observation of the entry site to ensure the balloon has not moved as its pumping characteristic varies according to its position in the aorta

(3) observation of the wound for sepsis

(4) reporting of excessive pain (the wound is not usually particularly uncomfortable);

(5) careful measurement of urine output and its quality; fluid balance is assessed

(6) observation of the limb distal to the balloon to watch for signs of occlusion, by comparing colour, pulses and difference in peripheral temperature in one limb compared to the other, and compared with the central core temperature

(7) patient's attitude and acceptance of the equipment.

Ancillary equipment

The effectiveness of the balloon pump is measured by various parameters, including haemodynamic studies and ECG, therefore several lines are attached to the patient from the pump itself and from separate pieces of equipment.

To assess *blood pressure* there will be: (*a*) an indwelling radial artery cannula; (*b*) a Swan Ganz catheter, or similar, for pulmonary artery pressure; and pulmonary wedge pressure (left atrial pressure). If thermodilution studies are performed to assess cardiac output a multiple lumen catheter is used. Cardiac output is sometimes determined by computer incorporated in the balloon pump machine.

Central venous line is attached to assess central venous pressure.

Blood pressure is checked manually from time to time and

blood gases are assessed regularly using blood taken from the radial arterial line.

To monitor the *cardiac rhythm* a second set of ECG electrodes may be attached which connect to the Unit's central monitoring system (see Chapter 3). The balloon pump machine may have a 'freeze' button on the cardioscope to study the trace.

Temperature is recorded using a peripheral probe attached to a foot and a rectal probe for core temperature.

A *temporary pacemaker* may be *in situ* also.

Post-operatively, or if the patient has respiratory problems, he may be intubated and connected to a *ventilator*.

Oxygen via a face mask or nasal cannulae is often given initially.

The nurses, medical staff and technicians are careful of all these attachments and extra equipment to ensure that tension is not applied inadvertently on any lines, causing them to disconnect or fall out. Strapping holding lines in place should be checked and renewed regularly. Use tape, pinned to the bedclothes, provided the patient is immobile, to relieve the weight of cables, or specially designed cable clips. Ensure electrical apparatus cannot be disconnected.

Nurse's role
To nurse a patient surrounded by so much equipment is demanding and rewarding. One, two or three nurses are assigned per shift to care for him.

To care for a patient adequately with an intra-aortic balloon pump the nurse should have a wide knowledge so that she will be able to continually assess her patient's condition from various observations, parameters measured, and results of tests. To be able to predict events and to inform her medical colleagues when problems occur, she must have a good working knowledge of: (*a*) anatomy, physiology of the cardiovascular, renal and pulmonary systems; (*b*) normal laboratory values and results of tests relating to these systems; (*c*) drugs used — their specific uses, side effects and interaction with other drugs.

The nurse should constantly observe all parameters so she can inform medical staff and technicians if changes occur beyond prearranged limits. If she is expected to perform certain tasks, such as increasing or decreasing an infusion rate should particular events occur, it is advisable that instructions are clearly and precisely written down by the doctor so there is no room for doubt.

Vital signs. Observations should be made of pulse rate, blood pressure, pulmonary artery pressure, pulmonary wedge pressure until stable. These should be made every quarter-hour initially, decreasing to every half-hour, then hourly.

Cardiac rhythm is observed constantly and assessed hourly. A 12 lead ECG should be taken if the rhythm changes. If the monitoring electrodes attached to the balloon pump need to be re-sited for any reason the technician should be informed as the balloon timing may need to be readjusted.

If the patient has a pacemaker the nurse should be familiar with its controls.

Urine output. Measure and record hourly. Specific gravity, osmolality, creatinine clearance and urine electrolytes (sodium and potassium) are checked regularly as well as routine ward testing.

Balloon pump equipment. Ensure there are sufficient materials and extra apparatus which may be needed, such as spare gas bottles. Inform the technician of alarms which cannot be corrected, changes in arterial wave form which may be related to the timing, changes in rhythm and dysrhythmias.

Ancillary equipment and attachments. An electrically-safe environment must be vigilantly ensured (see Chapter 8).

Infection. Protect the patient from infection. The entry site of the balloon should be dressed at least every other day and swabs taken regularly for bacterial culture. Note any discharge, swelling or redness. A groin wound is particularly susceptible to infection.

Diet. If the patient is able to eat he should have a light diet with salt restriction and carefully measured fluid intake. Constipation should be prevented by the usual methods used on the Unit, e.g. granules of bran to add bulk, or regular aperients.

Physiotherapy. Encourage the patient to move his toes and ankles and to bend the unaffected leg. The leg with the catheter must not be flexed at the groin. Arm, shoulder and neck movements are beneficial and regular chest physiotherapy is essential.

Supplies. Ensure there are sufficient supplies such as strapping, intra-venous equipment, manometer lines, oxygen.

Basic care of the patient, physically and mentally. As so many parameters are constantly measured the nurse must ensure the patient has time to rest. Tests are often carried out by staff from different departments who may not realize how often a patient is disturbed. They should be encouraged to come to the patient at specific times. By keeping a chart in view of every visit and time spent at the patient's bedside for a 24-hour period the nurse can help instill awareness into others.

The patient may choose to be kept in ignorance of the pump and other equipment but if he wishes to know about it care should be taken to explain its function according to his intellectual level. Patients quickly become used to the constant sound of the machine, a mere hum in modern pumps, and are only disturbed if it stops without warning for any reason.

Consideration for the patient's family and close friends. Lengthy explanations are sometimes needed to relieve relatives' anxieties and to put them into perspective. The time spent is rewarded as their more relaxed attitude is conveyed to the patient.

All the above factors are equally important in the management of the patient. The *senior nurse* should know what action to take in all eventualities. Many situations she can deal with herself but she must know when to call the physician, surgeon or technician. To help her, written guidelines and criteria regarding specific parameters should be given. These include: high and low blood pressure; orders for starting, increasing or decreasing infusion of drugs or volume expanders; high and low limits for pulmonary artery pressure and pulmonary wedge pressure; orders for diuretics or volume expanders; high and low limit of heart rate and rhythm changes and use of anti-dysrhythmic drugs or use of pacemaker if *in situ*; urinary output – lowest limit per hour and orders for diuretics and volume expanders; temperature – high and low limits and instructions for re-warming or cooling the patient.

Demarcation lines of responsibility are difficult at times but it should be possible to decide who is in charge of certain aspects of patient care. For example, in some Units only the doctor or blood technician takes blood samples while in others it is done by the nurse. Technicians are not given enough responsibility for equipment on some Units so that a heavier burden falls on the nurse.

Good communications are essential so that each person in the team knows what is expected of him and his colleagues. 'Grey areas' which arise can be discussed and decisions enacted.

The patient is nursed initially semi-recumbent or flat as he will be hypotensive. He should be turned from side to side gently every two hours but sitting up is inadvisable beyond 45 degrees if the femoral approach is used, as the tubing may occlude or be displaced. Vigorous activity is discouraged which may dislodge the balloon catheter or any of the other measuring devices. Mild sedation is advisable to help allay fears and distress but encouragement and general chat with the patient, if he is at all receptive, will play the most important part in relaxing him.

The balloon is usually *in situ* for about 48 hours but it may be needed for as long as a month, so nursing care must be stringent to prevent problems arising from enforced inactivity.

Anti-coagulation therapy is not necessary to prevent clots forming on the balloon as the material is antithrombogenic but sometimes it may be given as the patient is inactive to prevent deep venous thrombosis.

The pump
There are several machines available to operate an intra-aortic balloon pump. The controls vary and the display panels show differing parameters. Methods of automatic and manual balloon-filling vary a little, but instructions are printed and displayed clearly so there is a constant reminder. Familiarity with the particular machine used in a hospital helps the operator to cope with it easily in time, and responses often become automatic.

The machine is electrically operated from mains supply with a standby rechargeable battery which automatically functions for one to three hours in case of power failure. The battery is also useful when transferring a patient. Design of hospital and lifts must be mentioned at this point as it is important that a patient can be moved from a Unit to an operating theatre and vice versa without detaching the pumping machine. Arrangements have to be made occasionally to nurse patients in the recovery room of a theatre if there is insufficient space to move him.

Controls on the pump include timing adjustments for start of balloon inflation and deflation. Difficulties sometimes occur if a pacemaker is in use as the machine may pick up the pacing artefact as an R wave, as mentioned earlier.

Calibration controls are available for ECG and pressure tracings. If other equipment is used for measurements it should be calibrated to the same level as the pump, or differences taken into account. The displays are digital, or sometimes several analogue traces displayed in different colours, or a combination of the two. Heart rhythms and arterial pressure waves may be shown simultaneously with artefacts showing where inflation stops and starts.

Various safety factors are incorporated. There may be a panel which lights up to display such faults as: inoperable pump, high pressure, low pressure, high gas volume, high leak rate and loss of ECG. Immediate attention can then be given to the fault without wasting time looking for it.

Sometimes a leak occurs somewhere in the system so that a low pressure alarm occurs. Balloon pumping action is interrupted temporarily while more gas fills the balloon system, then the cycle is re-started. Leaks most commonly occur at the connection of the balloon catheter with the machine, but improved design is overcoming this problem. Cracks occasionally occur in the tubing leading to the balloon.

Fluid sometimes collects in the tubing leading from the pump to the balloon. It is cleaning solution pushed out of the machine and is unimportant except that it can be noisy. Lifting the tubing regularly helps it drain back into the machine or the tubing can be arranged so that gravity allows it to flow back.

Reasonable changes in rate and regularity will be accepted but if extra systolic activity is excessive a fail-safe system holds the balloon in permanent exhaust mode (empty) until normal rhythm is restored or the timing re-set to cope with it.

Also if no R wave is received because the electrode has fallen off, a fail-safe system will prevent over-inflation of the balloon. If the input from the arterial pressure line demonstrates systole without the machine having received an R wave it will exhaust, and activate audible and visual alarm signals.

Numerous other safety factors are incorporated into the design which is continuously improved and modified as more research is undertaken.

Weaning

Discontinuing balloon pumping may be decided for several reasons:
(1) the patient's condition improves so that he no longer needs the support
(2) ischaemia occurs in the leg
(3) an inoperable situation is shown on angiography, e.g. large akinetic left ventricle
(4) marked deterioration of the patient, which no longer justifies use of the pump.

When a decision is made to discontinue the action of the intra-aortic balloon pump it is withdrawn gradually.

Various supportive drugs are used in conjunction with the

balloon pump. They are mainly positive inotropic agents or pressors, e.g. adrenaline and dopamine. As the patient's condition improves the supportive drugs are gradually decreased while carefully assessing cardiac function so that circulation may be supported by balloon pump alone. If supportive drugs are still given, the dose is carefully titrated as the patient is weaned off the pump. The frequency of pumping is decreased from pumping during every diastolic phase (1:1) to 2:1, 4:1 and sometimes 8:1, holding each phase for a set length of time until it is considered that the pump is no longer needed to support the circulation. The process takes a few hours.

Removal of balloon
This is usually done in the ward. Aseptic technique is used. After removal of the balloon and before the artery is sutured the distal lumen is checked to ensure there is no occluding clot. If the artery is damaged a piece of vein may be grafted on to it. After suturing and dressing, the wound is observed daily for haemorrhage, haematoma and signs of sepsis, and redressed with an occlusive dressing.

Gradual increase in activity of the affected leg is encouraged and the patient sits up more. Check distal pulses, temperature and colour of the limb. Sutures are removed after seven to ten days.

After balloon removal close observation of vital signs is essential initially, until the patient's condition proves to be stable.

The medical team should again give the nurse definite guidelines and establish criteria similar to those used when the balloon was first inserted.

One important factor relating to the successful use of the aortic balloon pump is its availability at the time when it is needed. At present the machinery often has to be moved from one hospital to another, which takes time as well as risking damage. It is an expensive item to buy and to run but, as more information is given, the machine becomes more highly developed and as more doctors learn to use it, the intra-aortic balloon pump will, no doubt, prove its worth.

Further reading
Mechanical Support of the Failing Heart and Lungs. David
    Bregman. New York; Appleton-Century-Croft (1977).

8. Safety

Electrically operated equipment is frequently used in all areas of a hospital. Simple tests are performed in Out Patient Departments and, as a patient becomes more critically ill, he is surrounded by increasing banks of mains- or battery-operated instruments and machines.

Safety Committees function at international, national and local levels to ensure a minimum high standard of performance and to encourage the development of new techniques. Manufacturers adhere to definite safety codes when designing equipment; therefore safe working of individual instruments is guaranteed and they are usually delivered in perfect order. Technicians are responsible for ensuring that they are set up and used correctly and for instructing doctors, nurses and other medical personnel in their use.

Nurses who care for patients attached to such equipment should take every opportunity to familiarize themselves with its purpose, use of controls, measures to prevent malfunction, methods of recognizing when it operates wrongly and know who to inform should problems occur.

All medical staff have opportunities and a duty to protect their patients, colleagues and themselves from electrical hazards, and should report suspicious equipment to the appropriate department as a matter of urgency. A regular maintenance programme ensures such hazards are quickly noted and corrected.

The human body is protected from electrical shock by intact skin up to certain levels which vary slightly in individuals. Dry skin offers greater resistance (i.e. insulates more) than wet skin. The heart is particularly susceptible to electric shock as normal function relies on organized patterns of electricity to produce a regular stimulation to cause the heart to beat. Electric shock may derange the normal pattern of activation and lead to chaotic electrical activity known as ventricular fibrillation (see Fig. 4.2). Normally a large current is required to set off ventricular fibrillation but very little current is needed if the electrical source is in direct contact with the heart, i.e. if the heart is 'electrically exposed'. Direct lines that can take current to the heart from an external source include pacemaker wires and pressure manometer lines terminating in a chamber of the heart — all by-pass the electrical insulation of the skin.

Electrical equipment that presents a particular hazard to the patient and operator is the defibrillator. Chapter 4 deals with this and, as long as the simple rules of protection are followed, there should be no hazard.

External pacemaker units are a special source of danger to the patient if incorrectly used either in the wrong mode (e.g. at a fixed rate instead of 'on demand') or by not recognizing when there is malfunction. These subjects are dealt with in Chapter 5.

Intravenous fluids contain electrolytes and can act like conducting wires causing electricity to flow along the column of fluid. Blood, containing sodium, potassium and calcium ions, is another example of a potential fluid conductor. Perspiration also conducts electricity.

Patients in Intensive Care areas are particularly at risk from electrical hazard. The patient may lie on an electrically operated bed covered by a hypothermic blanket attached to a ventilator, intra-aortic balloon pump and cardiac monitor and with a pacemaker wire or pulmonary artery line passing directly into the heart.

Leakage current

This is an unfortunate term used to describe the normal phenomenon of current produced from all mains electrical equipment which flows to the casing, thence to the floor — or 'earth' via the earth lead of a plug.

Electric potential is measured in volts compared to earth, generally considered to have a voltage of zero. It may be greater than earth (plus) or less than earth (minus) and will try to get back to zero or earth to reach an equilibrium. If a person touches a live current source while standing on the ground the electricity will flow through his body as current travels from a higher level to a lower level.

Very little leakage current, if any, flows through the patient as long as the earth wire is intact. However, if the earth wire breaks the whole leakage current may flow through the patient to earth, causing a hazard.

Various methods are used to minimize this possibility, including electrically 'isolating' the patient. This is achieved by designing the instrument circuit so that the patient, power line and earth wires are separate. Three-pin plugs which include an earthing wire are often used in preference to two-pin plugs.

Battery-operated equipment does not present 'leakage' problems so it is considered safer to use in many instances such as monitoring cardiac rhythms using an electrode attached to a needle in direct contact with the heart during pericardial aspiration.

Nurses should recognize other potentially hazardous situations. If the earth wire fails on any piece of equipment such as an older style cardiac monitor, electrically operated bed, or image intensifier for fluoroscopy, leakage current will flow through other paths in contact with it, e.g. a nurse or technician, the patient's bed, the patient, or other equipment. If the current is great enough a nurse may feel it but normally it goes undetected as the equipment itself continues to function. Poor earthing could be indicated by increased interference on a cardiac monitor or interference on pressure monitoring equipment, for example.

The nurse should think of herself as part of the electrical environment surrounding the patient as she could act unwittingly as an electrical conductor completing an electrical circuit.

Here are two examples of hazards causing current to flow directly through the patient's heart.

(a) The patient has a pacemaker wire terminating in the right ventricle. The nurse places her hand on the image intensifier machine which is incorrectly earthed and, simultaneously, touches the pacemaker wire. Current will flow directly from the faulty machine through the nurse, along the pacing wire and into the heart.

(b) The patient has an intravenous infusion of normal saline leading to the pulmonary artery. The cardiac monitor to which he is attached is an old model and has an earth fault. While the nurse is touching against the cardiac monitor she adjusts the infusion where it enters the patient, causing a spillage of saline which comes into contact with her hand. The leakage current from the faulty monitor flows through the nurse, along the saline, directly to the heart.

Other electrical equipment likely to be used in the vicinity of a patient which may become a hazard if improperly earthed includes fan, X-ray machine, bedside lamp, television set, mains radio set, electric razor and vacuum cleaner.

It is recommended that all such equipment is correctly earthed in accordance with modern accepted standards. As much equipment as possible should be electrically isolated from the patient.

It is good practice for the nurse to ensure she is not in contact with electrical equipment while touching the patient.

Wiring

Split cable insulation may expose electrical wiring to allow direct contact with the live wire. Be aware of power cables running across the floor. Do not snag or catch them when moving beds, lockers, etc. Do not allow equipment to stand on cables. When lowering the back of a bed or using bedsides ensure cable, particularly from the cardiac monitor, will not be trapped, fracturing the outer casing.

Never remove plugs from sockets by pulling on the cable as this could give faulty connections. Broken plugs fail to insulate against shock. Loose exposed wires are a potential hazard.

Report any loose wires, frayed ends and fractures so that they can be corrected by a properly qualified person. Do not attempt temporary repairs.

Never rest containers of fluid on electrical apparatus where it may be knocked over and the contents spilled into the internal workings.

While at the bedside develop the habit of looking at all connections and wires so that it becomes as automatic as checking that the intravenous fluid line is running correctly.

Clean electrical equipment with anti-static spray or spirit which will evaporate rather than damp dusting with the possible risk of squeezing water inside. Cleaning jobs in Intensive Care areas should be done by specially instructed regular domestic workers. Vacuum cleaners or other electrical cleaning apparatus should only be used when the Unit is empty of patients to minimize the risk of electrical interference and mishaps.

Ensure that there are sufficient electrical socket outlets to avoid having to unplug pieces of equipment constantly, with the possible risk of unplugging a vital piece of equipment such as the ventilator. For extra security label the ventilator plug and intra-aortic balloon pump plug, particularly.

When setting up apparatus, switch on at the mains first before the apparatus, as this could help to avoid blowing a fuse. When electrical apparatus is no longer needed, switch it off at the apparatus before switching off at the mains. This also avoids false alarms where a power supply failure alarm is fitted.

As far as possible the same types of plugs and sockets should be used throughout the hospital to avoid the risks involved with using adaptors. Rubber watertight plugs are used with ventilators and other equipment where water is involved.

Equipment frequently used in one area should have sufficient length of cable to avoid using extension leads but not too long to cause problems of excess cable. If excess cable is coiled, use large loops to avoid fracturing the wires.

Education is the only real way of recognizing the potential electrical hazards and preventing them. To understand electrical problems in depth it is advisable to read a manual specifically designed to teach nurses and technicians how electricity works, the problems that arise and how they can be prevented.

Further reading

Using Electrically Operated Equipment Safely with the Monitored Cardiac Patient. Hewlett-Packard (1970). This is a manual especially written for nurses and is very clear and helpful.

Patient Safety. Application note AN 718. Hewlett-Packard (1971).

Electromedical instrumentation. P. Bergvelt. Techniques of Measurement in Medicine 2. Cambridge University Press (1970). A guide for medical personnel deals with this subject in depth.

Index